1574

MRI of the Brain I: Non-Neoplastic Disease

The Raven MRI Teaching File

Series Editors

Robert B. Lufkin
William G. Bradley, Jr.
Michael Brant-Zawadzki

MRI of the Brain I: Non-Neoplastic Disease
William G. Bradley, Jr. and Michael Brant-Zawadzki, Editors

MRI of the Brain II: Non-Neoplastic Disease
Michael Brant-Zawadzki and William G. Bradley, Jr., Editors

MRI of the Brain III: Neoplastic Disease
Anton N. Hasso, Editor

MRI of the Spine
Robert Quencer, Editor

MRI of the Head and Neck
Robert B. Lufkin and William N. Hanafee, Editors

MRI of the Musculoskeletal System
John V. Crues III, Editor

MRI of the Body
David D. Stark, Editor

MRI of the Cardiovascular System
Rod Pettigrew and Orest Boyko, Editors

Pediatric MRI
Rosalind Dietrich, Editor

MRI: Principles and Artifacts
Edward Hendrick, Editor

THE RAVEN MRI TEACHING FILE

MRI of the Brain I: Non-Neoplastic Disease

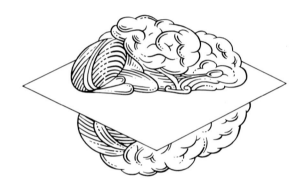

Editors

WILLIAM G. BRADLEY, JR., M.D., Ph.D.

Director of MRI and Radiology Research
Long Beach Memorial Medical Center
Long Beach, California

MICHAEL BRANT-ZAWADZKI, M.D., F.A.C.R.

Director of MRI
Hoag Memorial Hospital
Newport Beach, California

RAVEN PRESS NEW YORK

Raven Press, 1185 Avenue of the Americas, New York, New York 10036

Made in the United States of America

Library of Congress Cataloging-in-Publication Data

MRI of the brain: non-neoplastic disease/editors, William G.
  Bradley, Jr., Michael Brant-Zawadzki.
      p.   cm.—(The Raven MRI teaching file)
  Includes bibliographical references and index.
  ISBN 0-88167-745-0 (v. 1).—ISBN 0-88167-696-9 (v. 2)
  1. Brain—Magnetic resonance imaging.   I. Bradley, William G.
II. Brant-Zawadzki, Michael.   III. Series.
  [DNLM: 1. Brain Diseases—diagnosis.   2. Magnetic Resonance
Imaging.   WL 348 M939]
RC386.6.M34M76   1989
616.8′047548—dc20
DNLM/DLC
for Library of Congress   90-9107
                                                             CIP

The material contained in this volume was submitted as previously unpublished material, except in the instances in which credit has been given to the source from which some of the illustrative material was derived.

Great care has been taken to maintain the accuracy of the information contained in the volume. However, neither Raven Press nor the editors can be held responsible for errors or for any consequences arising from the use of the information contained herein.

Materials appearing in this book prepared by individuals as part of their official duties as U.S. Government employees are not covered by the above-mentioned copyright.

9 8 7 6 5 4 3 2 1

To our parents (who started it all):

William G. Bradley, Sr., M.D., Shirley A. Bradley, Michael Brant-Zawadzki, M.D., and Halina Brant-Zawadzki, M.D.

Magnetic Resonance Imaging (MRI) is a complex, rapidly evolving modality which has recently developed applications in all areas of diagnostic radiology. The successful radiologist in the 1990s *must* be proficient at MRI. To develop such proficiency is a formidable task, particularly for radiologists who were not exposed to MRI during their residencies. This 1,000 case MR teaching file is intended to help the practicing radiologist rapidly acquire a storehouse of experience which should aid development of proficiency in MRI. Cases have been carefully selected to show variable manifestations of common pathology as well as the occasional unusual case. The discussions have been kept brief, conforming to the teaching file format. If the reader focuses first on the left hand page while covering the right hand page, retention of information is significantly improved. Although the diagnosis in these workbooks is often suggested by the clinical history and presentation of selected images, the same information of the entire series is available in a convenient single video disk in which the reader is given the option to either choose the selected images reproduced in the printed workbooks or additional images including color and "movie" sequences from the complete imaging file. Additionally, the video disk format allows case presentation either with or without clinical information or orientation to a particular organ system. The video disk is available through Medical Interactive, 3708 Mt. Diablo Boulevard, Suite 120, Lafayette, California 94549.

The series editors would like to thank the section editors for their efforts in organizing the individual 100 case workbooks. This represents contributions from a large number of our friends and colleagues. This also allows us to show cases from a wide variety of manufacturers, MR instruments using a range of magnetic field strengths. We would also like to thank Mary Rogers and her staff at Raven Press for all their help and encouragement during the course of this project.

Robert B. Lufkin, M.D.
William G. Bradley, Jr., M.D., Ph.D.
Michael Brant-Zawadzki, M.D., F.A.C.R.

Volumes I and II of the Raven MRI Teaching File focus on non-neoplastic diseases of the brain. Volume I focuses on flow phenomena, vascular abnormalities, hemorrhage, and trauma, while Volume II focuses on hydrocephalus, infarction, and demyelinating disease. Although these topics are emphasized and thus provide some differentiation of Volumes I and II, in general, they should be taken together as there is considerable overlap.

The cases in these volumes are arranged in order and should be approached in sequence. The reader will get the most out of each case if the key images and history are reviewed on the left hand page prior to reading the diagnosis and discussion on the right hand page.

William G. Bradley, Jr., M.D., Ph.D.
Michael Brant-Zawadzki, M.D., F.A.C.R.

Acknowledgments

Cases in both volumes have come from high field and mid field systems at Hoag and Huntington, as well as from the systems of many of our colleagues who have either sent us interesting cases or asked us for a second opinion. We thank them for allowing us to use their cases in this teaching file series. We also thank those who have been indispensable in putting this teaching file together. At Huntington these were the 1989–1990 MR Fellows, Stephen Davis, M.D. and Louis Teresi, M.D.; technologists, Leslee Watson, Jose Jimenez, Laurel Adler, and Sheri Gregory. We thank Denise Longpre for manuscript preparation and Kaye Finley for everything else.

At Hoag, we thank, in particular, Janet Arnds for manuscript preparation, Jim Walling, Debbie Norman, Susan Steward, Jackie Oldeck, Kevin O'Brien who helped in case procurement and aides Arik Killion and Micah Eaton who helped with case selection. Without their efforts, this task would have been much more onerous.

THE RAVEN MRI TEACHING FILE

MRI of the Brain I: Non-Neoplastic Disease

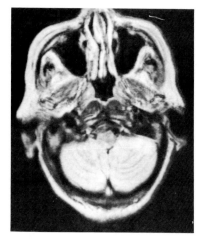

FIG. 1A. SE 3,000/40.

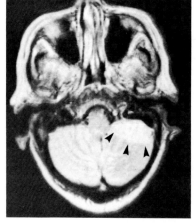

FIG. 1B. SE 3,000/40.

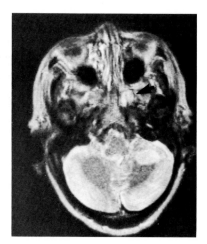

FIG. 1C. SE 3,000/80.

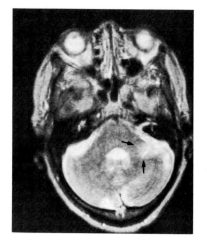

FIG. 1D. SE 3,000/80.

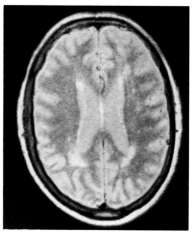

FIG. 1E. SE 3,000/40.

Clinical History

A 75-year-old man with sudden onset of vertigo and left hearing loss.

Findings

Axial 5 mm T2-W (SE 3,000/40 and 80) images are presented. There is a cortically based area of increased signal intensity involving the anterior inferior left cerebellar hemisphere (Figs. 1A–D). The anterior petrosal surface of the inferior hemisphere is completely involved (Figs. 1A and B). The lesion extends superiorly into the inferior lateral pons and the middle cerebellar peduncle (Fig. 1D, *black arrows*) and also involves the flocculus. Lesions 5–8 mm in diameter are present in the inferior left basal ganglia and bilaterally in the belly of the pons. There are multiple foci of increased signal intensity bilaterally in the periventricular regions (Fig. 1E). Mucus is noted in the lateral recess of the left sphenoid sinus (Fig. 1C, *black arrow*).

Diagnosis

Infarction in the distribution of the anterior inferior cerebellar artery, deep white matter infarcts, and small basal ganglia and pontine lacunae.

Discussion

An anterior inferior cerebellar artery territory infarct is the rarest of cerebellar infarcts. The distribution shown in this patient is typical. Of note is the characteristic convex posterior surface (Fig. 1B, *arrowheads*) delineating this vascular territory from that of the posterior inferior cerebellar artery (PICA). These two vessels share a variable amount of the inferior cerebellar hemisphere, although the PICA usually predominates. Lateral inferior pontine syndromes are commonly associated (Fig. 1D, *arrows*), and these give rise to ipsilateral deafness, tinnitis, and ataxia (as seen in this patient), as well as ipsilateral facial paralysis, impaired sensation, diplopia, and contralateral impaired pain and temperature sense to the body.

Fluid in the inferior recess of the sphenoid air sinus is common and should not be confused with an infratemporal fossa lesion.

Reference

1. Savoiardo M, Bracchi M, Passerini A, et al. The vascular territories in the cerebellum and brainstem: CT and MR studies, *AJNR* 1987;8:199–209.

Submitted by: Stephen J. Davis, M.D. and Louis M. Teresi, M.D., Huntington Medical Research Institutes, Pasadena, California; William G. Bradley, Jr., M.D., Ph.D., Senior Editor.

Study One

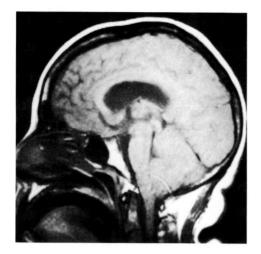

FIG. 2A. SE 600/20.

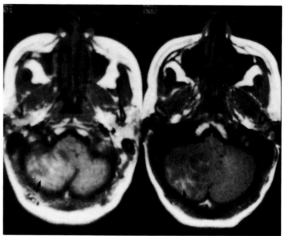

FIG. 2B. SE 600/20.

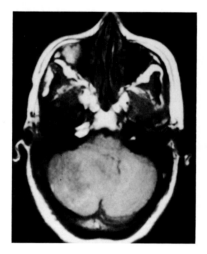

FIG. 2C. SE 600/20.

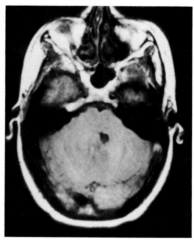

FIG. 2D. SE 600/20.

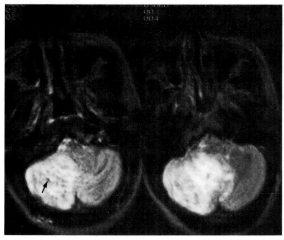
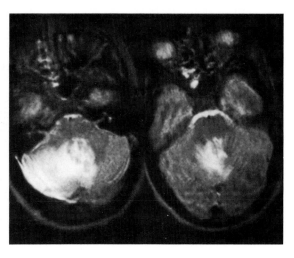

FIG. 2E. SE 2,800/80.   FIG. 2F. SE 2,800/80.

Study Two (3 months later)

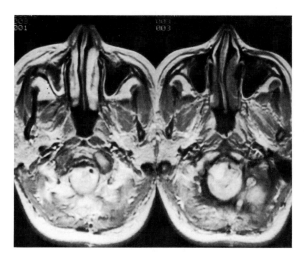
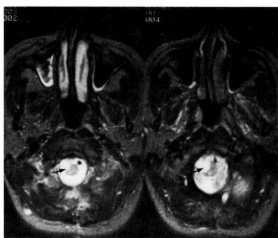

FIG. 2G. SE 2,800/30.   FIG. 2H. SE 2,800/80.

5

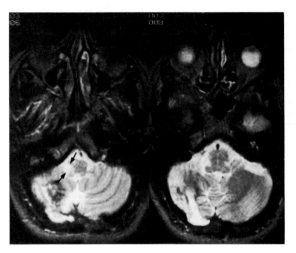

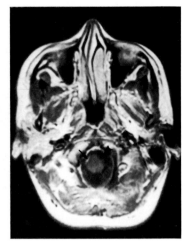

FIG. 2I. SE 2,800/80.   FIG. 2J. SE 600/20.   FIG. 2K. SE 600/20.

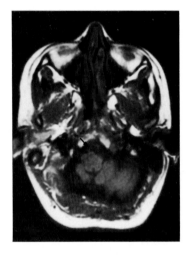

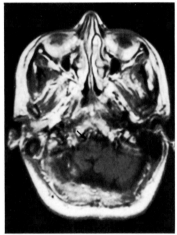

FIG. 2L. SE 600/20.   FIG. 2M. SE 600/20.

Clinical History

A 33-year-old woman who developed sudden onset of unsteady gait seven days prior to the initial scan, followed by a gradual onset of headaches and vomiting, then progressive lethargy, which developed over the next three days.

Findings

Axial and sagittal 5 mm T1-W (SE 600/20) and axial 5 mm T2-W (SE 2,800/30 and 80) images from the time of presentation are presented. A second set of images taken three months later includes axial 5 mm T2-W (SE 2,800/30 and 80) and axial 5 mm pre- and post-gadolinium T1-W (SE 600/20) images. On the initial study, there is a large cortically based lesion involving the inferior right cerebellar hemisphere and adjacent vermis (Figs. 2E and F). There is evidence of hemorrhage, with ribbons of T1 shortening in the cerebellar cortex causing increased signal on the T1-weighted sequence (Fig. 2B, *black arrows*) and similar cortically based ribbons of T2 shortening noted inferiorly in the cerebellar hemisphere on the T2-weighted sequence (Fig. 2E, *black arrow*). There is considerable associated mass effect with swelling of the cerebellum, compression, and displacement of the 4th ventricle, compression of the medulla and lower pons, and secondary obstructive hydrocephalus (Figs. 2A, C, and D). There is a rim of high signal intensity surrounding the lateral ventricles. The T2-weighted scans are degraded by patient motion due to the patient's obtunded condition.

Images from the second study show resolution of the posterior fossa mass effect and the obstructive hydrocephalus and resolution of the methemoglobin on the pre-contrast T1-weighted image. There is persistence of gyriform T2 shortening in the inferior cerebellar hemisphere, indicating hemosiderin deposition (Fig. 2I). There is evidence of infarction involving the lateral aspect of the right medulla (Fig. 2I, *black arrows*). This lesion extends into the anterolateral aspect of the upper cervical cord (Fig. 2H, *black arrows*). On none of the images is the left vertebral artery clearly seen, and there is serpiginous contrast enhancement in the line of the left vertebral artery (Figs. 2K and M, *black arrows*) when compared with the pre-gadolinium study, in which there is some increase in intensity in the line of this vessel (Figs. 2J and L, *black arrows*). This is in contrast to the flow void seen in the right vertebral artery (Fig. 2K, *arrowhead*), indicating patency of this vessel. A right posterior fossa craniotomy has been performed between the two studies, and there are some residual changes associated with this (Fig. 2I).

Diagnosis

Hemorrhagic infarction in the distribution of the posterior inferior cerebellar artery and contrast enhancement of the right vertebral artery.

Discussion

The initial films show features typical of hemorrhagic infarction in the posterior inferior cerebellar artery (PICA) distribution with considerable associated mass effect and secondary obstructive hydrocephalus. The second set of images shows evidence of associated infarction of the lateral medulla. The lateral medullary syndrome (Wallenberg's syndrome) is sometimes associated with PICA distribution infarcts, usually due to thrombosis of the vertebral artery. The short medullary artery supplying the lateral medulla originates more often from the distal vertebral artery but may originate from the PICA or, less often, from the anterior inferior cerebral artery or proximal basilar artery. In this case, there is evidence of occlusion of the right vertebral artery, and the contrast enhancement within the artery is likely to be due to either enhancement in the wall secondary to repair of an acute spontaneous dissection or enhancement of evolving thrombosis within this vessel. Given the patient's age, spontaneous dissection of the vertebral artery would seem a strong possibility as the original diagnosis in this patient.

The lateral medullary syndrome (Wallenberg's syndrome) presents acutely with vertigo, vomiting, ipsilateral facial pain, and dysphagia, and shows ipsilateral palatal paralysis, Horner's syndrome, pain and temperature loss in the ipsilateral face, and contralateral body and cerebellar signs in the limbs.

Reference

1. Savoiardo M, Bracchi M, Passerini A, et al. The vascular territories in the cerebellum and brainstem: CT and MR studies. *AJNR* 1987;8:199–209.

Submitted by: Stephen J. Davis, M.D. and Louis M. Teresi, M.D., Huntington Medical Research Institutes, Pasadena, California; William G. Bradley, Jr., M.D., Ph.D., Senior Editor.

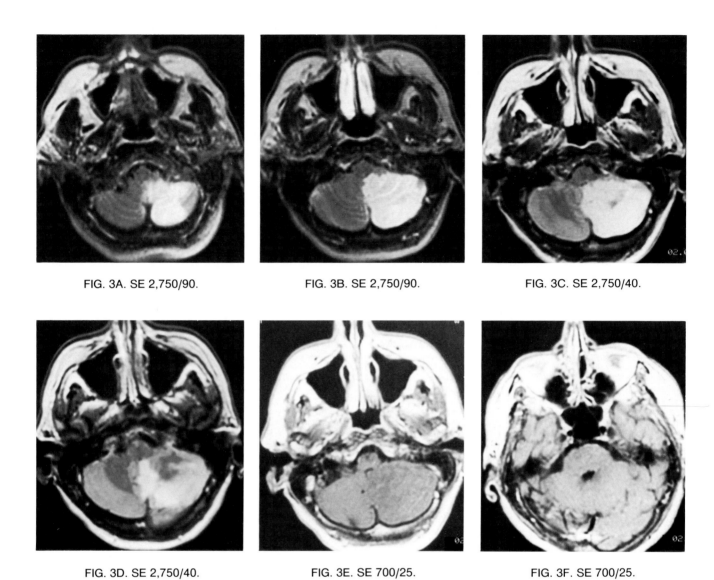

FIG. 3A. SE 2,750/90.   FIG. 3B. SE 2,750/90.   FIG. 3C. SE 2,750/40.

FIG. 3D. SE 2,750/40.   FIG. 3E. SE 700/25.   FIG. 3F. SE 700/25.

Clinical History

Sudden onset four days previously of ataxia with vomiting and nausea.

Findings

Axial 5 mm T2-W (SE 2,750/40 and 90) and axial 5 mm post-gadolinium T1-W (SE 700/25) images are presented.

The inferior half of the left cerebellar hemisphere shows increased signal intensity on the T2-weighted sequences (Figs. 3A–D) and mild decreased signal on T1-weighted (Fig. 3E) images. The lesion is cortically based and involves the whole inferior posterior surface of the cerebellar hemisphere and adjacent inferior vermis. More superiorly, it spares the anterior left cerebellar hemisphere and most of the white matter of the brachium pontis. The lesion does not extend to the superior cerebellar surface.

There is considerable swelling of the left cerebellar hemisphere with compression of the 4th ventricle, which is also "rotated" forward (Figs. 3E and F). There is no evidence of contrast enhancement following gadolinium administration (Figs. 3E and F) or of obstructive hydrocephalus. The lateral medulla is not involved.

Prominent perivascular spaces are incidentally noted adjacent to the basal ganglia, near the vertex, and in the deep white matter.

Diagnosis

Acute infarction in the distribution of the posterior inferior cerebellar artery (PICA).

Discussion

The features typical of acute infarctions are shown with increased signal on T2-weighted sequences, with minimal decrease in signal on T1-weighted images, and with mass effect in the absence of contrast enhancement. The distribution of this lesion is typical of the PICA. The region supplied by this artery is variable, but it typically encompasses the inferior posterior surface of the cerebellar hemisphere and ipsilateral inferior vermis. The posterior limit is at the level of the great horizontal fissure. The lateral angle (is the watershed region between the PICA and the anterior inferior cerebellar artery (AICA). The AICA typically involves the whole anterior petrosal cerebellar hemisphere. The deep white matter of the cerebellum is typically supplied by the superior cerebellar artery, which also supplies the whole superior aspect of the cerebellar hemisphere and ipsilateral superior vermis. The mass effect is usually seen between days 3 and 10. Larger posterior fossa infarcts may cause severe secondary deterioration from brainstem compression or secondary aqueductal obstruction.

Reference

1. Savoiardo M, Bracchi M, Passerini A, et al. The vascular territories in the cerebellum and brainstem: CT and MR studies. *AJNR* 1987;8:199–209.

Submitted by: Stephen J. Davis, M.D. and Louis M. Teresi, M.D., Huntington Medical Research Institutes, Pasadena, California; William G. Bradley, Jr., M.D., Ph.D., Senior Editor.

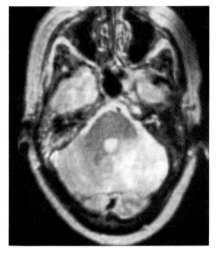

FIG. 4A. SE 3,000/80.

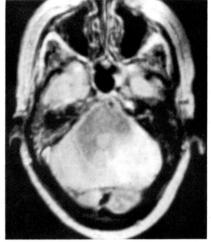

FIG. 4B. SE 3,000/40.

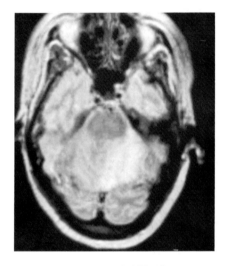

FIG. 4C. SE 3,000/40.

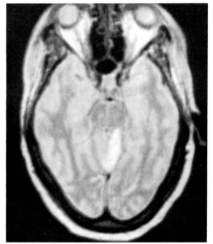

FIG. 4D. SE 3,000/40.

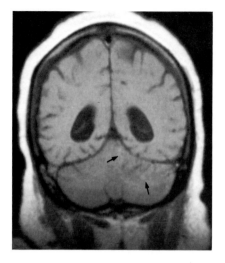
FIG. 4E. SE 500/30.

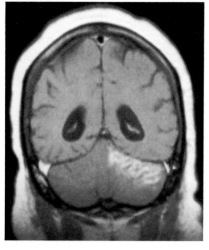
FIG. 4F. SE 500/30 with Gd-DTPA.

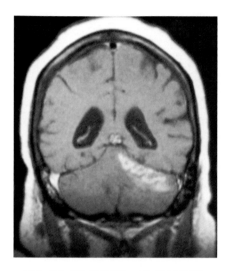
FIG. 4G. SE 500/30 with Gd-DTPA.

Clinical History

A 66-year-old woman with sudden onset of headache, dizziness, vomiting, and gait disturbance 12 days prior to this scan.

Findings

Axial 5 mm T2-W (SE 3,000/40 and 80), pre-gadolinium coronal T1-W (SE 500/30), and post-gadolinium coronal and axial T1-W (SE 500/30) images are presented.

On the T2-weighted sequences, there is a cortically based diffuse increase in signal intensity involving the superior half of the left cerebellum. This is associated with mild mass effect, with slight displacement of the rostral and mid pons toward the right and slight effacement of the superior 4th ventricle (Figs. 4A–D). There is a slight gyriform increase in signal intensity in this region on the T1-weighted pre-contrast scan (Fig. 4E, *black arrows*). Following gadolinium administration, there is diffuse gyriform cortical enhancement along the cerebellar folia of the superior half of the left cerebellar hemisphere (Figs. 4F–J). Lesions 5 mm in diameter are noted on the T2-weighted sequences involving the left caudate nucleus and the left thalamus, and there are scattered punctate foci of increased intensity in the deep white matter. Mucosal thickening is noted in the right mastoid air cells.

Diagnosis

Subacute left superior cerebellar infarct, left caudate and thalamic lacunae, mild deep white matter ischemic changes, and right mastoiditis.

Discussion

Subacute cerebellar infarcts are characterized by contrast enhancement and mild mass effect. Although enhancement of an infarct has been seen in the laboratory within 24 hours of vascular occlusion, clinically it is not usually seen before seven days. It may persist for six to eight weeks. Contrast enhancement is due to leak of gadolinium DTPA across the immature blood-brain barrier of the proliferating capillaries that are found at the edge of infarcts. It characteristically produces irregular serpiginous patterns following the cortical surface of lobar infarcts, such as in this case. Enhancement peaks in approximately two weeks and is likely to be due to a combination of loss of autoregulation leading to arteriovenous shunting and "luxury perfusion," blood-brain barrier breakdown, and neovascularity in active gliosis. Lacunar infarcts enhance around the periphery and may simulate other ring-enhancing lesions, such as infections or tumors. The central necrotic area of infarcts does not enhance. In the clinical setting of multiple brain infarcts, contrast enhancement may help to distinguish chronic infarcts from more recent events. Contrast-enhanced scans performed two weeks post-ictus will help to separate subacute from more chronic lesions in the context of multiple lesions.

The mass effect of posterior fossa infarction, seen predominantly between days 3 and 10, may result in significant compression of brainstem structures, causing secondary deterioration. Obstructive hydrocephalus occurs in up to 15% of cases. The extent of mass effect is determined by the size of the infarct and is caused by cytotoxic edema and breakdown of the blood-brain barrier with leakage of proteinaceous fluid into the interstitial space.

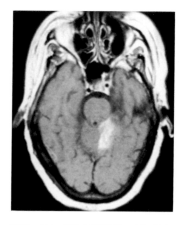 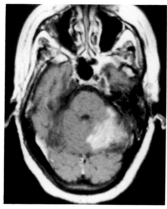 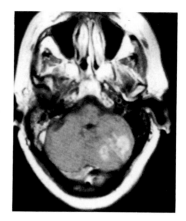

FIG. 4H. SE 500/30 with Gd-DTPA. FIG. 4I. SE 500/30 with Gd-DTPA. FIG. 4J. SE 500/30 with Gd-DTPA.

References

1. Djang WT, Drayer BP. Posterior fossa: occlusive vascular disease. In: Taveras J, Ferrucci J, eds. *Radiology diagnosis—imaging and intervention,* vol. 3, Ch. 71. Philadelphia: JB Lippincott, 1986.
2. Imakita S, Nishimura T, Naito H, et al. Magnetic resonance imaging of human cerebral infarction: enhancement with Gd-DTPA. *Neuroradiology* 1987;29:422–429.
3. Virapongse, Mancuso A, Quisling R. Human brain infarcts: Gd DTPA-enhanced MR imaging. *Radiology* 1986;161:785–794.

Submitted by: Stephen J. Davis, M.D. and Louis M. Teresi, M.D., Huntington Medical Research Institutes, Pasadena, California; William G. Bradley, Jr., M.D., Ph.D., Senior Editor.

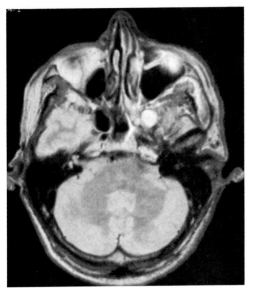

FIG. 5A. SE 3,000/40.

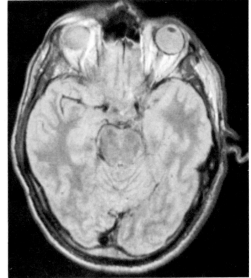

FIG. 5B. SE 3,000/40.

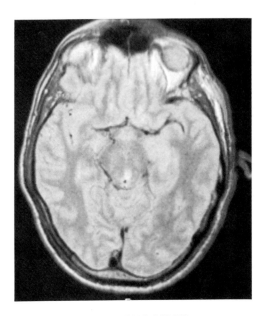

FIG. 5C. SE 3,000/40.

Clinical History

A 57-year-old man with left 3rd nerve palsy with pupillary sparing.

Findings

Axial 5 mm T2-W (SE 3,000/40) images are presented.

There is a 4 × 8 mm lesion involving the left 3rd nerve nucleus in the midbrain, sharply demarcated in the midline from a normal-appearing right-sided posterior tegmentum of the midbrain (Fig. 5C). There is no evidence of associated obstruction of the aqueduct.

Incidentally noted is mucus in the left sphenoid (Fig. 5A) and posterior ethmoidal air cells, mucoperiosteal thickening in the remainder of the ethmoids, and prominent Virchow-Robin spaces near the vertex.

Diagnosis

Midbrain infarct.

Discussion

Localized extraocular palsy may result from "surgical" mass lesions (usually with involvement of the pupillary response), such as cerebral tumors or aneurysms of the circle of Willis, or from medical lesions (usually with pupillary sparing), such as diabetes mellitus, multiple sclerosis, polyarteritis, sarcoid, syphilis, meningitis, and arteriosclerosis.

The configuration of this lesion strongly suggests infarction involving the paramedian perforating branches of the thalamoperforate arteries, which originate from the tip of the basilar artery and from the adjacent interpeduncular pre-communicating segments of the posterior cerebral arteries. These vessels supply the medial one-third of the midbrain tegmentum and cerebral peduncle (paramedian branches). The lateral two-thirds of the tegmentum and most of the cerebral peduncle are supplied by short circumferential branches arising from the posterior communicating arteries, while the remaining tectum is supplied by the long circumferential arteries arising from the posterior cerebral artery and the superior cerebellar arteries. Infarcts involving this region may extend into the inferior thalamus.

The sharp demarcation in the midline is characteristic of midbrain infarction. The main differential diagnosis is multiple sclerosis; however, at follow-up one year later, there was slight resolution of the ocular palsy and no other evidence of multiple sclerosis. A larger lesion at this site, which extends forward to involve the cerebral peduncle and therefore gives rise to a contralateral hemiparesis, is termed "Weber's syndrome." More extensive infarction that includes the medial lemniscus and red nucleus causes contralateral hemianesthesia and choreiform motions and is termed "Benedikt's syndrome."

Reference

1. Djang WT, Drayer BP. Posterior fossa: occlusive vascular disease. In: Taveras J, Ferrucci J, eds. *Radiology diagnosis—imaging and intervention,* vol. 3, Ch. 71. Philadelphia: JB Lippincott, 1986.

Submitted by: Stephen J. Davis, M.D. and Louis M. Teresi, M.D., Huntington Medical Research Institutes, Pasadena, California; William G. Bradley, Jr., M.D., Ph.D., Senior Editor.

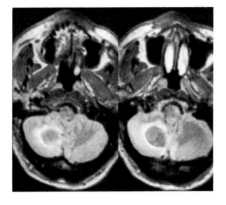

FIG. 6A. SE 3,000/40.

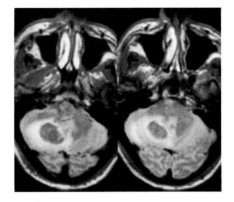

FIG. 6B. SE 3,000/40.

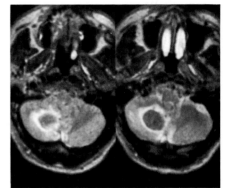

FIG. 6C. SE 3,000/80.

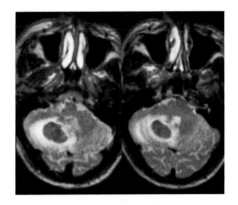

FIG. 6D. SE 3,000/80.

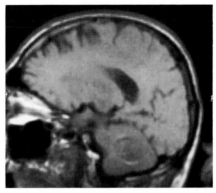

FIG. 6E. SE 500/40.

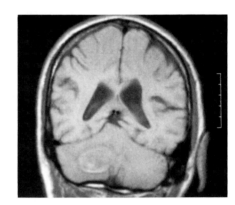

FIG. 6F. SE 500/30.

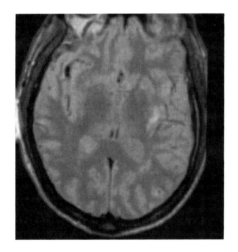

FIG. 6G. SE 3,000/40.

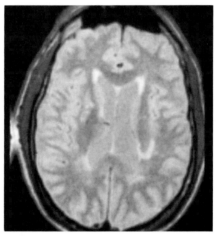

FIG. 6H. SE 3,000/40.

Clinical History

A 62-year-old man with sudden on-set 48 hours previously of dizziness, nausea, vomiting, headache, and speech difficulty. Long-standing hypertension. Right cerebellar signs on examination.

Findings

Axial 5 mm T2-W (SE 3,000/40 and 80), coronal 10 mm T1-W (SE 500/30), and sagittal 5 mm T1-W (SE 500/40) images are presented.

There is a 3 cm diameter well-circumscribed lesion in the right cerebellar hemisphere that has a central area of increasingly low signal intensity as the TE is lengthened, typical of T2 shortening effect (Figs. 6A–D). This central region is hypointense on a T1-weighted image (Fig. 6E) and is surrounded by a thin rim of high signal intensity (Fig. 6F), indicating T1 shortening. This rim is also seen on the T2-weighted sequences (Figs. 6A–D), where there is, in addition to the focal rim, a more diffuse surrounding high signal intensity, consistent with edema. There is considerable mass effect from this lesion, with displacement of the 4th ventricle to the left and effacement of the overlying cerebellar sulci. No associated abnormal vessels are seen.

There is a 3 × 15 mm lesion involving the posterior left putamen and adjacent external capsule (Fig. 6G) and a second lesion of similar size involving the posterior left corona radiata (Fig. 6H), representing lacunar infarcts. There are several punctate foci of high signal intensity in the deep white matter bilaterally (Fig. 6I). Mild prominence of the cerebral sulci and lateral ventricles is consistent with mild cortical atrophy.

Diagnosis

Three-centimeter acute–early subacute right cerebellar hematoma, lacunar infarcts, and ischemic changes in the periventricular white matter.

Discussion

Acute hematomas are characterized by a central low intensity on T2-weighted images, with T2 shortening caused by the magnetic susceptibility effect of deoxyhemoglobin in red blood cells. As shown in this case, this effect occurs at midfield (0.35 T), although it is more obvious with high-field strength scanners. There is a rim of methemoglobin surrounding the lesion, best seen on the T1-weighted images, causing increased signal intensity from T1 shortening due to the paramagnetic effects of methemoglobin. As in this case, methemoglobin typically forms in the periphery of a hematoma and then extends inward with time. Surrounding this is some edema adjacent to the hematoma, causing T2 lengthening.

Hemorrhage at this site is a well-recognized complication of hypertension. In order of frequency, hypertensive bleeds involve the basal ganglia, thalamus, pons, and cerebellum.

Reference

1. Gomori JM, Grossman RI. Mechanisms responsible for the appearance and evolution of intracranial hemorrhage. *Radiographics* 1988;8:427–451.

Submitted by: Stephen J. Davis, M.D. and Louis M. Teresi, M.D., Huntington Medical Research Institutes, Pasadena, California; William G. Bradley, Jr., M.D., Ph.D., Senior Editor.

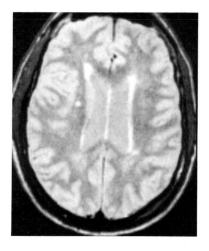

FIG. 6I. SE 3,000/40.

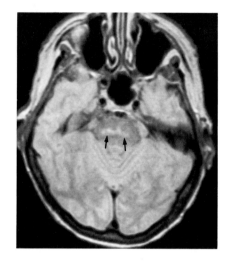

FIG. 7A. SE 3,000/40.

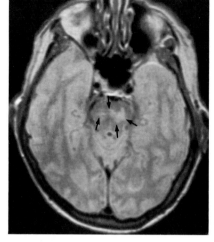

FIG. 7B. SE 3,000/40.

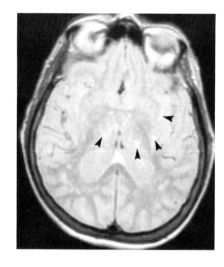

FIG. 7C. SE 3,000/40.

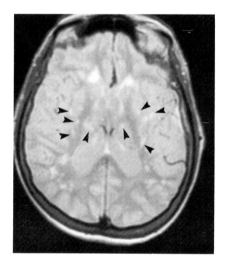

FIG. 7D. SE 3,000/40.

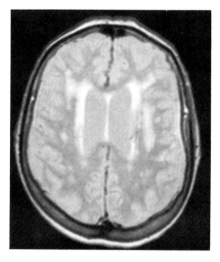

FIG. 7E. SE 3,000/40.

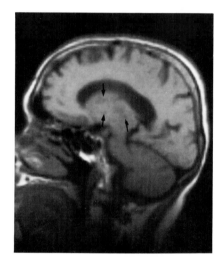

FIG. 7F. SE 500/40.

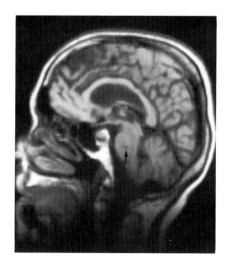

FIG. 7G. SE 500/40.

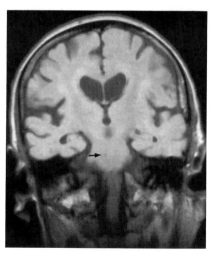

FIG. 7H. SE 1,000/30.

Clinical History

An 85-year-old woman with a sudden onset, three days prior to scan, of staggering to the left, with balance defect and nausea.

18

Findings

Axial 5 mm T2-W (SE 3,000/40), sagittal 5 mm T1-W (SE 500/40), and coronal 1 cm (SE 1,000/30) images are presented. There is an irregular area of increased signal intensity on T2-weighted images measuring approximately 5 × 20 mm in size traversing the midpons (Figs. 7A and B, *arrows*). This is larger on the left side, where it measures approximately 10 mm (Fig. 7B). No lesion is present in the medulla or midbrain, and there is no MR evidence of hemorrhage or mass effect. The major cerebral arteries are intact.

Multiple punctate and confluent areas of increased signal intensity are present in the periventricular white matter bilaterally (Fig. 7E). There are also multiple punctate 3–5 mm lesions in the lentiform nuclei, thalami, and posterior limbs of the internal capsules bilaterally (Figs. 7C and D, *arrowheads*). Punctate foci of low signal intensity are seen in this region on the T1-weighted images (Fig. 7F, *arrows*). There is a 3 mm focus of decreased signal intensity in the right side of the midpons (Figs. 7G and H, *black arrows*).

Diagnosis

Lacunar infarcts bilaterally in the pons and basal ganglia and deep white matter infarcts.

Discussion

Lacunar infarcts are small, deep cerebral infarcts usually encountered in the setting of hypertension resulting from occlusion of small penetrating arteries. These include small lenticulostriate branches of the anterior and middle cerebral arteries, thalamoperforating branches of the posterior cerebral arteries, and paramedial branches of the basilar artery. Most of these have no distal anastamoses, and many are single unbranched vessels. Pathologically, these small vessels are subject to lipohyalinosis, affecting arteries less than 200 μm in diameter and causing lacunae ranging from 3 to 7 mm in size. Microatheromatous disease occludes slightly larger vessels, particularly in the lenticulostriate distribution, and results in larger lacunae. As in this case, lacunae occur predominantly in the basal ganglia, internal capsule, thalamus, and brainstem.

The brainstem lesions characteristically are confined to the central portions of the mid- and upper pons, with sparing of the medulla, midbrain, and cerebellar peduncles, and there is usually no evidence of signal alteration on T1-weighted sequences. The great majority of patients with pontine findings on MR images have no clinical evidence of brainstem infarction. In this patient, the size of the left-sided pontine lesion may account for her balance deficit and nausea, a clinically manifest pontine infarction. Clinically significant pontine infarcts are more likely to be localized to one side of the brainstem and have a paramedian distribution, a relative sagittal orientation, and evidence of T1 lengthening. Such T1 prolongation may distinguish infarction from less clinically significant gliosis in which the T1 is normal.

References

1. Brown JJ, Hesselink JR, Rothrock JF. MR and CT of lacunar infarct. *AJNR* 1988;9:477–482.
2. Salomon A, Yeats AE, Burger PC, Heinz ER. Subcortical arteriosclerotic encephalopathy: brainstem findings with MR imaging. *Radiology* 1987;165:625–629.
3. Perret J, Hommell M, Pollak, et al. Clinical and radiological correlations in ischaemic brainstem infarcts: a magnetic resonance imaging study. In: Gouaze A, Salamon G, eds. *Brain anatomy and magnetic resonance imaging.* Berlin: Springer-Verlag, 1988.

Submitted by: Stephen J. Davis, M.D. and Louis M. Teresi, M.D., Huntington Medical Research Institutes, Pasadena, California; William G. Bradley, Jr., M.D., Ph.D., Senior Editor.

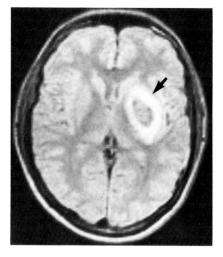

FIG. 8A. SE 2,000/28.

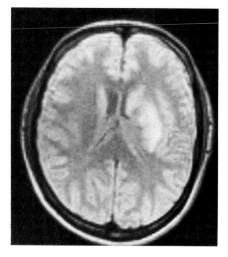

FIG. 8B. SE 2,000/28.

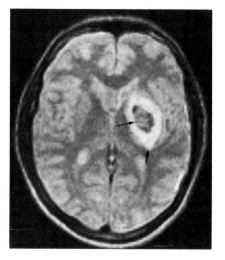

FIG. 8C. SE 2,000/56.

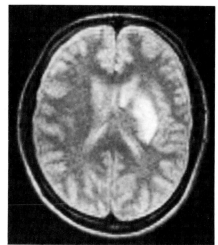

FIG. 8D. SE 2,000/56.

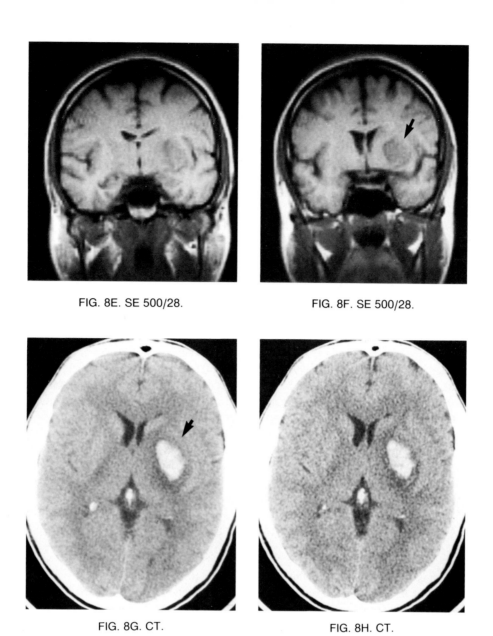

FIG. 8E. SE 500/28.   FIG. 8F. SE 500/28.

FIG. 8G. CT.   FIG. 8H. CT.

Clinical History

A 35-year-old man with renal failure and hypertension with acute onset of right-sided weakness.

Findings

Axial T2-W (SE 2,000/28 and 56) and coronal T1-W (SE 500/28) images and a non-contrast CT scan are provided for review. The axial SE 2,000/28 images show a lesion in the left basal ganglia (Fig. 8A, *arrow*). The lesion has a low-signal center and a high-signal periphery. On the SE 2,000/56 images, the low-signal center becomes more hypointense (Fig. 8C, *long arrow*), whereas the high-signal periphery is unchanged (Fig. 8C, *short arrow*). The coronal T1-weighted images show that the lesion is slightly hypointense to surrounding brain and has a nearly uniform signal (Fig. 8F, *arrow*), unlike that seen on the T2-weighted images. The axial CT scan shows the lesion as high density surrounded by a region of lower density (Fig. 8G, *arrow*).

Diagnosis

Acute basal ganglia hemorrhage.

Discussion

The findings in this case are consistent with an acute hemorrhage. The high-density center on the CT scan corresponds to the low-signal region on the T2-weighted images, representing extravasated blood. The low-density periphery of the lesion on the CT scan corresponds to the high-signal region on the T2-weighted images, representing edema.

Review of the appearance of hemorrhage on MRI. Hematoma evolution on MR displays all the major paramagnetic iron-containing compounds in an orderly and concentric fashion. Intracerebral hematomas can be staged as hyperacute, acute, early subacute, late subacute, and chronic. The exact time frame of these changes is approximate; however, the sequence of pathologic and MR changes is characteristic (Table 1).

A hyperacute hematoma is seen in the first few hours after blood extravasation, before the plasma is resorbed and before the conversion of oxyhemoglobin to deoxyhemoglobin. Oxyhemoglobin has no unpaired electrons and, thus, is not paramagnetic. Therefore, hyperacute hematomas behave like a simple protein solution. They will be hypointense to isointense on T1-weighted images and hyperintense to isointense on proton density and T2-weighted images.

Acute hematomas are less than one week old. Within hours, the plasma fraction of hemorrhage is resorbed, raising the hematocrit of the hematoma to approximately 90%. Concurrently, the hemoglobin, which is deprived of oxygen because it is sequestered, becomes deoxygenated to its deoxyhemoglobin state. Deoxyhemoglobin is paramagnetic; it has four unpaired electrons. Although its unpaired electrons are inaccessible to water protons for a dipole to dipole interaction (to cause T1 shortening), intracellular deoxyhemoglobin results in heterogeneous magnetic susceptibility in the retracted clot. When an external magnetic field is applied, the higher susceptibility inside the red blood cell containing the deoxyhemoglobin results in a field gradient across the cell membrane. Although the spin-echo sequence will correct for static field inhomogeneities, it will not completely correct for the effects of water proton diffusion across field gradients. On spin-echo sequences, the T2 relaxation rate (1/T2) due to intracellular deoxyhemoglobin increases as the square of the magnetic field strength and increases with lengthening of the interecho interval. The increased relaxation rate (shortened T2) results in a decrease in the signal intensity of acute hemorrhage on T2-weighted images at mid- to high field. Acute hemorrhages are isointense or slightly hypointense to gray matter on T1-weighted and proton density weighted images. Surrounding edema appears hyperintense on T2-weighted and proton density images and isointense or mildly hypointense to gray matter on T1-weighted images.

The subacute stage begins after approximately one week. The deoxyhemoglobin is converted to methemoglobin, initially in the hematoma periphery. The *in vivo* auto-oxidation of oxyhemoglobin to methemoglobin is an incompletely understood complex process, but some statements can be made from empirical observations at this time. Some oxygen is needed to oxidize the heme iron to the ferric form, yet normal levels of oxygen allow the methemoglobin reductase systems to reduce it back to the ferrous form. Methemoglobin formation thus appears to occur most rapidly when there is a small amount of oxygen available. For these reasons, the interface between normal parenchyma and the hematoma periphery is the favored site for methemoglobin formation. It is in this location that deoxyhemoglobin and the oxidizing agents necessary for the formation of methemoglobin are optimally found.

Methemoglobin is paramagnetic: it has five unpaired electrons. These electrons are accessible to water protons for dipole to dipole interactions, which shorten T1. This effect is not significantly affected by field strength or cell integrity. Intracellular methemoglobin also leads to heterogenous magnetic susceptibility, which increases with the square of the magnetic field and is responsible for the short T2 and persistent low signal on T2-weighted images in early subacute hemorrhages.

Thus, early subacute hematomas (approximately one week old) demonstrate a peripheral ring of variable hyperintensity on T1-weighted images and hypointensity on T2-weighted images. Further hypointensity occurs with longer interecho intervals and higher fields.

During the following few weeks, the hyperintensity on T1-weighted images extends to fill the entire hematoma. This is due to the progressive conversion of deoxyhemoglobin to methemoglobin. During the late subacute phase, these areas also become hyperintense on proton density and T2-weighted images at all field strengths. This is due to red blood cell lysis resulting in free methemoglobin, which is hyperintense on all image pulse sequences due to dipole to dipole interactions no longer opposed by susceptibility effects.

The chronic stage is defined by the presence of a hemo-siderin rim. In order for this to occur, the peripheral red blood cells must have lysed and thus appear hyperintense on all image pulse sequences due to free methemoglobin. This appearance may persist for months to years. Reactive macrophages that migrate to the hematoma periphery digest the hemoglobin products and deposit insoluble hemosiderin granules in their lysosomes. These hemosiderin-laden macrophages are not removed from the brain (they are removed to some extent in most other tissues) and persist indefinitely in the hematoma periphery. After approximately one week, in the cerebral parenchyma immediately adjacent to the hematoma, there appears a ring of marked hypointensity on T2-weighted images with a long interecho interval at high field, which is mildly hypointense on T1-weighted and proton density-weighted images, corresponding to hemosiderin-laden macrophages. This is due to the superparamagnetic qualities of hemosiderin: its T2 relaxation rate increases quadratically with field strength and with lengthening of the spin-echo interecho interval.

TABLE 1. *MR appearance of intraparenchymal hematomas*

Stage	Time	Compartment	Hemoglobin	Intensity	
				T1-W	T2-W
Hyperacute	<24 hours	Intracellular	Oxyhemoglobin	iso → hypo	iso → hyper
Acute	1–3 days	Intracellular	Deoxyhemoglobin	iso	hypo
Subacute					
Early	3+ days	Intracellular	Methemoglobin	hyper	hypo
Late	7+ days	Extracellular	Methemoglobin	hyper	hyper
Chronic	14+ days				
Center		Extracellular	Hemichromes	iso → hypo	iso → hyper
Rim		Intracellular	Hemosiderin	hypo	hypo

(Modified from Bradley and Bydder [2].)
Abbreviations: iso, isointense; hypo, hypointense; hyper, hyperintense.

References

1. Gomori JM, Grossman RI. Mechanisms responsible for the appearance and evolution of intracranial hemorrhage. *Radiographics* 1988;8:427–451.
2. Bradley WG. Hemorrhage. In: Bradley WG, Bydder G, eds. *MRI atlas of the brain.* New York: Raven Press/London: Martin Dunitz, 1990;205.
3. Clark RA, Watanabe AT, Bradley WG, Roberts JD. Acute hematomas: effects of deoxygenation, hematocrit, and fibrin-clot formation and retraction on T2 shortening. *Radiology* 1990;174:201–206.
4. Bradley WG, Schmidt PG. Effect of methemoglobin formation on the MR appearance of subarachnoid hemorrhage. *Radiology* 1985;156:99–103.

Submitted by: Louis M. Teresi, M.D. and Stephen J. Davis, M.D., Huntington Medical Research Institutes, Pasadena, California; William G. Bradley, Jr., M.D., Ph.D., Senior Editor.

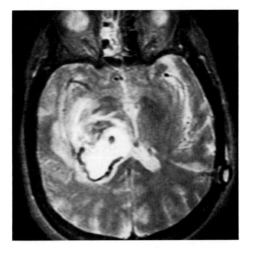

FIG. 9A. July 11, 1988, SE 2,800/70.

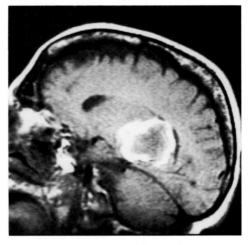

FIG. 9B. July 11, 1988, SE 600/20.

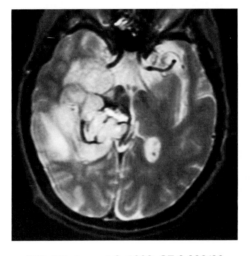

FIG. 9C. August 3, 1988, SE 2,800/80.

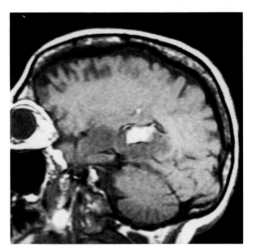

FIG. 9D. August 3, 1988, SE 600/20.

Clinical History

A 60-year-old woman with a sudden change in mental status and left-sided weakness.

Findings

The axial T2-weighted image reveals a high-signal mass centered in the region of the right ventricular trigone, with a peripheral low-signal border. A T1-weighted sagittal image (Fig. 9B) reveals elevated signal intensity within the mass seen just above the tentorium in the right posterior temporal region. Images obtained eight weeks later show a decreasing hemorrhagic component within the core of the lesion, but progressive mass in the more anterior deep temporal lobe both on the T2-weighted (Fig. 9C) and T1-weighted (Fig. 9D) images.

Diagnosis

Pathologic hemorrhage, malignant glioma.

Discussion

Although it is tempting to assign the cause of a spontaneous hemorrhage to hypertension or another cause of hemorrhagic strokes, such as occult vascular malformations, several criteria can be helpful in differentiating these entities. Neoplasms often show surrounding edema, whereas acute focal hemorrhage is generally unassociated with significant edema. Obviously, in cases of metastatic disease, multiplicity is a strong clue. In this case, the presence of the low signal border in the hemorrhage suggests an episode of previous bleeding. Although this is nonspecific and can obviously occur with occult arteriovenous malformation, the possibility of a pathologic focus is raised.

References

1. Sze G, Krol G, Olsen WL, et al. Hemorrhagic neoplasms: MR mimics of occult vascular malformations. *Am J Radiol* 1987;149:1223–1230.
2. Atlas SW, Grossman RI, Gomori JM, et al. Hemorrhagic intracranial malignant neoplasms: spin echo MR imaging. *Radiology* 1987;164:71–77.

Submitted by: Michael Brant-Zawadzki, M.D., Senior Editor.

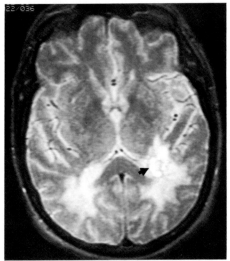

FIG. 10A. SE 2,800/70.

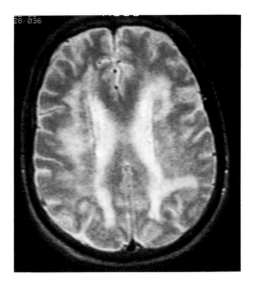

FIG. 10B. SE 2,800/70.

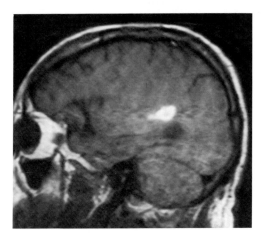

FIG. 10C. SE 600/20.

Clinical History

A 57-year-old man brought to the emergency room comatose. Blood pressure was 250/150.

Findings

The axial T2-weighted images (Figs. 10A and B) revealed diffuse high-signal abnormalities in the deep periventricular white matter. Note the relative small size of the ventricular system (Fig. 10A). Also, a curvilinear region of strikingly high signal intensity is seen immediately at the left ventricular trigone (Fig. 10A, *arrow*). This region corresponds to the high-signal abnormality on the T1-weighted sagittal image (Fig. 10C).

Diagnosis

Hypertensive encephalopathy, with focal hemorrhage.

Discussion

This patient shows the typical findings of the "breakthrough" edema of hypertensive encephalopathy. This is due to the extravasation of fluid and proteins across the blood-brain barrier when the thresholds of cerebral autoregulation have been breached by the high level of systemic blood pressure achieved in such patients. Not surprisingly, hemorrhages can accompany such episodes, as in this case. The appearance of this diffuse white matter change and the presence of small ventricular size (reflecting the increased intracranial pressure) in the setting of acutely elevated blood pressure fits very well with the diagnosis. The rapidity with which the patient's blood pressure rises and the degree of elevation relative to the patient's baseline blood pressure are the two most important factors responsible for the development of hypertensive encephalopathy.

References

1. Houser RA, Lacey M, Knight MR. Hypertensive encephalopathy: magnetic resonance imaging demonstration of reversible cortical and white matter lesions. *Arch Neurol* 1988;45:1078–1083.
2. Rail DL, Perkin GD. Computerized tomographic appearance of hypertensive encephalopathy. *Arch Neurol* 1980;37:310–311.

Submitted by: Michael Brant-Zawadzki, M.D., Senior Editor.

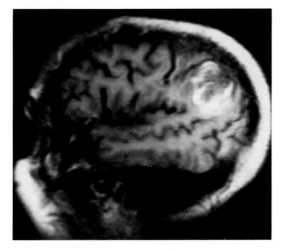

FIG. 11A. SE 800/20.

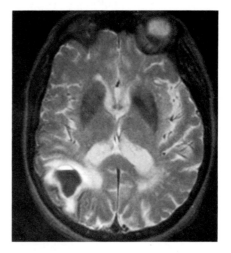

FIG. 11B. SE 2,800/70.

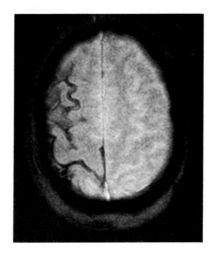

FIG. 11C. SE 75/20.

Clinical History

A 77-year-old woman with a previous right hemispheric hemorrhage, now with sudden onset of confusion and mild left weakness.

Findings

The T1-weighted sagittal sequence (Fig. 11A) shows an irregularly shaped lesion with high signal intensity characteristics in the periphery. The T2-weighted axial scan of this lesion shows a predominantly low signal intensity core, with a cap of high signal intensity surrounded by edema of the white matter (Fig. 11B). Mild mass effect is apparent.

The highest axial slice, a GRASS sequence (Fig. 11C), shows a serpentine area of signal loss throughout the high parietal cortex.

Diagnosis

Spontaneous intracerebral hemorrhage, repeat episode.

Discussion

The lower parietal, acute lesion is quite typical for a recent parenchymal hemorrhage. The lesion's low signal intensity on the T2-weighted sequences is attributable to a combination of magnetic susceptibility effects accentuated by the high field (1.5 T) of the instrument used and the increased hematocrit as well as increased protein content of the retracted fibrin clot. The small high-signal cap most likely represents methemoglobin in solution, the methemoglobin having been converted from the deoxyhemoglobin responsible for the magnetic susceptibility effect in the lower portion of the lesion. The methemoglobin is also responsible for the bright signal intensity on the T1-weighted image in the periphery. Note that these components are easily separable from the surrounding vasogenic edema of the white matter.

The high serpentine sulcal pattern of low signal intensity on the gradient echo sequence is quite typical for siderosis-hemosiderin deposition over the convexity of the brain, most likely related to the hemorrhagic stroke this patient suffered two years previously.

The occurrence of repeated hemorrhages in the brain without underlying pathology (tumor, infection) is most often seen in patients with hypertension. In this particular case, the patient was not hypertensive. Brain biopsies showed amyloid angiopathy. Amyloid angiopathy is seen in 5–10% of all patients over the age of 65 years and produces friability of the smaller perforating vessels. Repeated brain hemorrhages can occur in patients so affected. A differential diagnosis for recurrent brain hemorrhages, in addition to tumor, is venous thromboses (possibly due to sagittal sinus thrombosis) or vasculitis. Younger patients with such episodes should be investigated for the presence of basilar vascular occlusive disease (moyamoya).

References

1. Case C. Intracerebral hemorrhage: nonhypertensive causes. *Stroke* 1986;17:590–598.
2. Tyler K, et al. Cerebral amyloid angiopathy with multiple intracerebral hemorrhages. *J Neurosurg* 1982;57:286–289.
3. Gomori J, et al. Intracranial hemotomas: imaging by high-field MR. *Radiology* 1985;157:87–92.

Submitted by: Michael Brant-Zawadzki, M.D., Senior Editor.

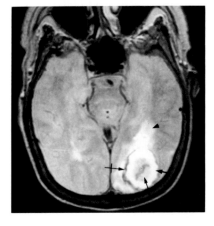
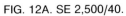

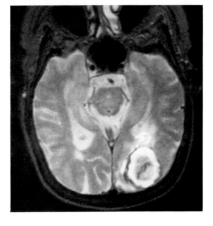

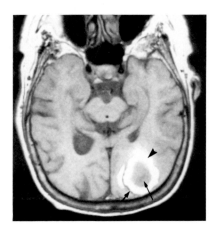

FIG. 12A. SE 2,500/40.

FIG. 12B. SE 2,500/80.

FIG. 12C. SE 600/25.

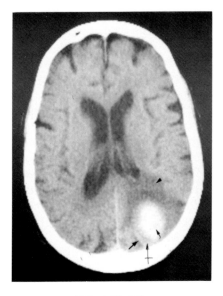

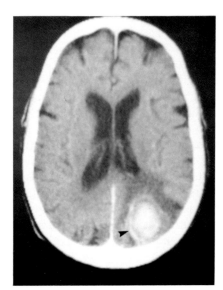

FIG. 12D. CT.

FIG. 12E. CT with contrast.

Clinical History

An 84-year-old demented woman complaining of problems with vision.

Findings

Axial T2-W (SE 2,500/40 and 80) and axial T1-W (SE 600/25) images and non-enhanced and enhanced CT scans are provided for review. The axial SE 2,500/40 image shows a lesion in the left parietal-occipital lobe. The center of the lesion is somewhat heterogeneous and isointense to gray matter (Fig. 12A, *long arrow*). The isointense center is surrounded by a region of hyperintensity (Fig. 12A, *short arrow*) that, in turn, is surrounded by a thin rim of hypointensity (Fig. 12A, *crossed arrow*). High intensity spreads in an irregular fashion from the lesion anteriorly (Fig. 12A, *arrowhead*). The appearance of the lesion is similar on the axial SE 2,500/80 image (Fig. 12B). The axial SE 600/25 image shows that the center of the lesion remains isointense to brain (Fig. 12C, *long arrow*) and that the high-intensity peripheral ring (Fig. 12C, *arrowhead*) corresponds to the region of hyperintensity seen on the SE 2,500/40 and 80 images (Fig. 12A, *short arrow*). The thin hypointense rim around the lesion (Fig. 12A, *crossed arrow*) is less conspicuous on the SE 600/25 image (Fig. 12C, *short arrow*). Similarly, the irregularly shaped high-signal region anterior to the lesion (Fig. 12A, *arrowhead*) is also less conspicuous.

The non-enhanced CT scan shows a high-density lesion (Fig. 12D, *long arrow*) surrounded by a low-density region (Fig. 12D, *crossed arrow*), further surrounded by a high-density rim (Fig. 12D, *short arrow*). Low density extends anteriorly from the lesion (Fig. 12D, *arrowhead*). The contrast-enhanced CT scan shows that the high-density rim enhances (Fig. 12E, *arrowhead*), whereas the high-density center and low-density surrounding rim do not enhance.

Diagnosis

Hyperacute hemorrhage within late subacute-chronic hemorrhage.

Discussion

The findings in this case are most consistent with a "hyperacute" hemorrhage within a prior "late subacute" hemorrhage (Table 1, Case 8). The high-density center on the CT images corresponds to isointense regions on both T1- and T2-weighted images, reflecting oxyhemoglobin in freshly extravasated blood. The low-density material surrounding the high-density center corresponds to hyperintensity on the T1- and T2-weighted images, reflecting extracellular methemoglobin in a prior hemorrhage.

The age and clinical presentation of this patient, as well as the location of the hemorrhage, is suggestive of amyloid angiopathy. Amyloid angiopathy is a frequent cause of nonhypertensive hemorrhage in older persons. Over the age of 70 years, more than 40% of brains reviewed in one autopsy series demonstrated the presence of amyloid in the cerebral parenchymal blood vessels. Between the ages of 60 and 70, only approximately 12% of brains demonstrated amyloid change in the blood vessels. This disease affects only the arterioles of the cortex. The media and adventitia are infiltrated and replaced by amyloid, and elastic lamina may become fragmented, split, or destroyed. Segmental fibrinoid degeneration, hyalin, and obliterative changes and microaneurysms may develop. This vascular disease has not been found in the white matter, basal ganglia, brainstem, or cerebellum. The cortical arterioles are most frequently involved in the parietal region.

The patients commonly have dementia and, pathologically, Alzheimer's plaques may be found in association with the vascular lesions. The angiopathy, however, is often present in the absence of Alzheimer's changes or clinical dementia. The amyloid change is probably not related to a specific disease entity, but rather is due to age-related change in the blood vessels. The hemorrhage associated with amyloid angiopathy primarily involves the cortex with irregular borders, surrounding edema, and frequent extension into the adjacent portion of the brain. This is in contrast to the usual deep ganglionic location of hypertensive hemorrhages, which only occasionally extend to the brain surface.

Reference

1. Vinters HV, Gilbert JJ. Amyloid angiopathy: its incidence and complications in the aging brain. *Stroke* 1981;12:118.

Submitted by: Louis M. Teresi, M.D., Stephen J. Davis, M.D., and Mark Ziemba, M.D., Huntington Medical Research Institutes, Pasadena, California; William G. Bradley, Jr., M.D., Ph.D., Senior Editor.

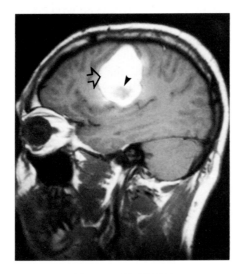

FIG. 13A. SE 600/20.

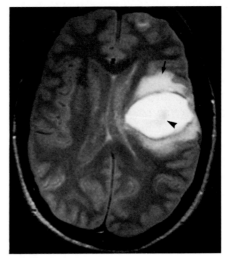

FIG. 13B. SE 2,700/30.

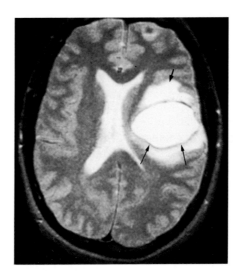

FIG. 13C. SE 2,700/80.

Clinical History

A 35-year-old man without significant past medical history, presenting with acute right arm and leg weakness.

Findings

Axial T2-W (SE 2,700/30 and 80) and sagittal T1-W (SE 600/20) images are provided for review. The sagittal SE 600/20 image shows a high-signal mass in the left parietal lobe in the region of the primary sensory and motor strips (Fig. 13A, *open arrow*). The high signal within the mass persists on the SE 2,700/30 and SE 2,700/80 axial images, which also show a thin rim of hypointensity surrounding the mass (Figs. 13B and C); this is most pronounced on the SE 2,700/80 image (Fig. 13C, *long arrows*). Hyperintensity suggestive of edema is also seen around the mass on the SE 2,700/80 sequence (Fig. 13C, *short arrow*).

In the center of the mass there is a region of isointensity, seen best on the SE 600/25 sagittal image (Fig. 13A, *arrowhead*). On the SE 2,700/30 sequence, this region is faintly visible (Fig. 13B, *arrowhead*), and it is not seen on the more T2-W SE 2,700/80 sequence (Fig. 13C).

Diagnosis

Persistent oxyhemoglobin within late subacute hematoma.

Discussion

This case illustrates some of the difficulties in interpreting MR images of a hemorrhage. Although the center of this lesion is isointense on the T1-weighted image, it becomes *hyperintense* on the T2-weighted images, like a protein solution. This has been postulated to be another appearance of hyperacute hemorrhage (oxyhemoglobin). This is particularly true when the center of large hematomas remains liquid as clot retraction, per se, leads to T2 shortening.

Lobar intracerebral hemorrhages consist of bleeding peripheral to the basal ganglia and thalami. They comprise 10–32% of nontraumatic cerebral hemorrhages. A wide variety of etiologies account for lobar intracerebral hemorrhage, including aneurysms, arteriovenous malformations (AVMs), anticoagulant therapy, neoplasm, bleeding diatheses, and microaneurysms associated with systemic hypertension or vasculitis.

Arteriovenous malformations present primarily either as seizure or hemorrhage. The first hemorrhage occurs most frequently in the second to fourth decades of life, and recurrent hemorrhage is most common in the fourth to sixth decades. The smaller the lesion, the greater the risk of hemorrhage. Thus, large intraparenchymal hemorrhages may obscure the underlying AVMs.

Another cause of lobar intracerebral hemorrhage is a peripheral aneurysm. It is estimated that 4% of aneurysms are peripheral (unrelated to the circle of Willis or horizontal segment of the middle cerebral artery). The majority are located in the middle cerebral artery branches and are usually mycotic in etiology, often associated with bacterial endocarditis.

Cerebral amyloid angiopathy is a cause of spontaneous intracerebral hemorrhage in the elderly population. The hemorrhage usually involves the parieto-occipital area and tends to be superficial. Atraumatic spontaneous intracerebral hemorrhage in a normotensive elderly patient should arouse the suspicion of amyloid angiopathy.

Hypertensive hemorrhage usually occurs in the putamen, thalamus, and cerebellum, with the putamen being the most common site. Lobar intracerebral hemorrhage associated with amphetamine abuse has been described. This is secondary to necrotizing angitis with microaneurysm formation.

In the relatively young patient in this case, the primary considerations for the cause of his intracerebral hemorrhage would be AVM, aneurysm, vasculitis, and bleeding diathesis.

Reference

1. Ropper AH, Davis KR. Lobar cerebral hemorrhage: acute clinical syndromes in 26 cases. *Ann Neurol* 1980;8:141–147.

Submitted by: Louis M. Teresi, M.D., Stephen J. Davis, M.D., and Mark Ziemba, M.D., Huntington Medical Research Institutes, Pasadena, California; William G. Bradley, Jr., M.D., Ph.D., Senior Editor.

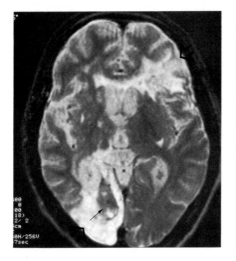 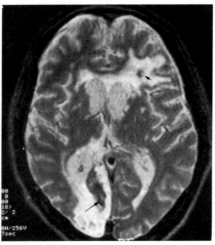

FIG. 14A. SE 2,600/100.   FIG. 14B. SE 2,600/100.

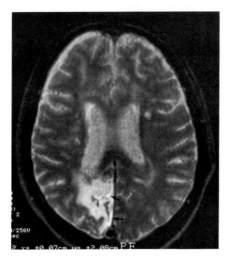 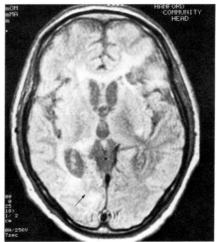

FIG. 14C. SE 2,600/100.   FIG. 14D. SE 2,600/25.

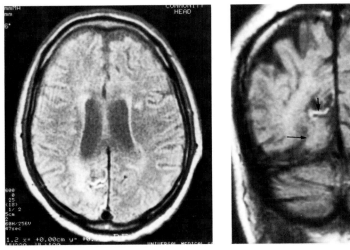

FIG. 14E. SE 2,600/25.

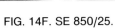

FIG. 14F. SE 850/25.

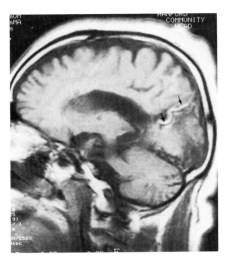

FIG. 14G. SE 600/25.

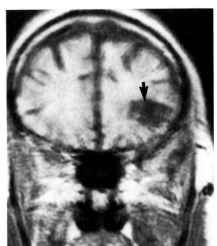

FIG. 14H. SE 850/25.

Clinical History

A 63-year-old man with acute onset of left homonymous hemianopia.

Findings

Axial T2-W (SE 2,600/25 and 100), coronal T1-W (SE 850/25), and sagittal T1-W (SE 600/25) images are provided for review. The axial SE 2,600/100 sequence shows two large regions of hyperintensity: one within the occipital lobe on the right and the second in the left frontoparietal lobe on the left (Fig. 14A, *open arrows*). Regions of hypo- to isointensity are noted in the occipital (Figs. 14A and B, *long arrows*), and frontoparietal (Fig. 14B, *short arrow*) hyperintense regions, which are isointense on the 2,600/25 sequence (Fig. 14D, *arrow*). The region of hypo- to isointensity on the SE 2,600/100 sequence in the right occipital lobe is isointense with brain on the SE 850/25 image (Fig. 14F, *long arrow*). The similar smaller region of hypo- to isointensity in the left frontoparietal lobe is not seen in the large region of hypointensity on the coronal SE 850/25 sequence (Fig. 14H, *arrow*).

A gyriform region of hyperintensity is seen in the calcarine cortex on the SE 2,600/100 and 25 sequences (Fig. 14C, *arrows*), which is high signal on the T1-W (SE 850/25 and SE 600/25) images (Figs. 14F and G, *short arrows*).

Diagnosis

Acute hemorrhagic infarctions of the right occipital and left frontoparietal lobes and late subacute hemorrhage in the right calcarine cortex. The left frontoparietal lesion is in a watershed distribution, whereas the right occipital lesion is in the distribution of the right posterior cerebral artery.

Discussion

The region of hypo- to isointensity on the SE 2,600/100 sequence, which is isointense to brain on the T1-weighted image, corresponds to a region of acute hemorrhage, the signal intensity being secondary to intracellular deoxyhemoglobin (Table 1, Case 8). With intracellular deoxyhemoglobin, one usually sees at least some hypointensity on a SE 2,600/25 image and, in this case, the SE 2,600/25 image shows the region of hemorrhage as isointense. This is consistent with the preferential T2-shortening characteristics of deoxyhemoglobin, which are more pronounced on long TE images and at high field. The images in this case were acquired on a 0.5-T imager; thus, the T2 shortening produced by deoxyhemoglobin will not be accentuated, although one would still expect to see some T2 shortening on a SE 2,600/25 sequence. The logical conclusion is that the images were acquired at the transition from hyperacute to acute hemorrhage (an "early acute" hemorrhage); thus, reflecting signal characteristics of nonparamagnetic oxyhemoglobin intermixed with a small amount of deoxyhemoglobin. The gyriform region of increased signal intensity on the SE 2,600/25 and 100 and SE 600/25 sequences in the calcarine cortex is consistent with late subacute hemorrhage (i.e., extracellular methemoglobin, which is high signal on T1- and T2-weighted images).

Acute hemorrhagic cortical infarctions are less hypointense on T2-weighted images at high field strengths than intracerebral hematomas of the same age. This appears to be due to higher local oxygen tension secondary to the hyperemia of the early revascularization and luxury perfusion associated with hemorrhagic cortical infarctions. This higher oxygen tension and pH lowers the concentration of intracellular deoxyhemoglobin. This increases the T2 relaxation time, which is proportional to the square of the intracellular deoxyhemoglobin concentration.

Hemorrhage is the hallmark of embolic infarction and is found when ischemic infarction is followed by reperfusion, usually when an embolus has fragmented. Hemorrhagic cortical infarctions also tend to occur in watershed zones and may occur at the margin of bland cortical infarction. They have a predilection for the deeper cortical layers and the deepest gyral infoldings. Due to the frequently petechial nature of hemorrhagic cortical infarctions, there may be no true hematoma center or periphery. Therefore, hemosiderin deposits may occur in the same distribution as the acute hemorrhages. At times, one may not be able to use location or morphology to differentiate the hypointensity on T2-weighted images of intracellular deoxyhemoglobin from that of hemosiderin deposits. However, the deoxyhemoglobin of acute hemorrhage is associated with edema (high intensity on T2-weighted images) and sulcal effacement, whereas the hemosiderin of chronic infarct is associated with atrophy and gliosis (high intensity on T2-weighted images), causing prominent sulci.

References

1. Hecht-Leavitt C, Gomori JM, Grossman RI, et al. High-field MR imaging of hemorrhagic cortical infarction. *AJNR* 1986;7:587–594.
2. Davis KR, Ackerman RH, Kistler JP, et al. Computed tomography of cerebral infarction: hemorrhagic, contrast enhancement and time of appearance. *Comput Tomogr* 1977;1:71–76.

Submitted by: Louis M. Teresi, M.D., Stephen J. Davis, M.D., and Mark Ziemba, M.D., Huntington Medical Research Institutes, Pasadena, California; William G. Bradley, Jr., M.D., Ph.D., Senior Editor.

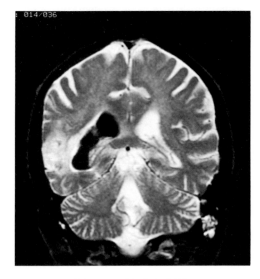

FIG. 15A. SE 2,800/90.

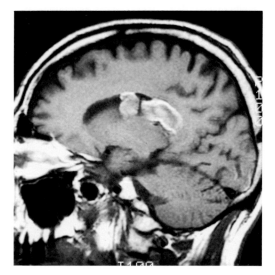

FIG. 15B. SE 600/20.

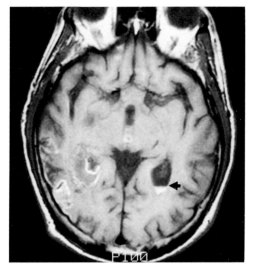

FIG. 15C. SE 800/20.

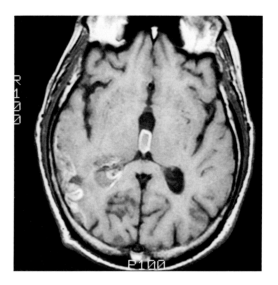

FIG. 15D. SE 800/20.

Clinical History

A 72-year-old man, three weeks post-right temporal infarct, with a sudden change in consciousness.

Findings

The coronal T2-weighted image shows a striking decrease in signal intensity within the posterior right lateral ventricle and proximal temporal horn. Associated with this is elevation of signal intensity in the right posterior temporal lobe (Fig. 15A). The sagittal T1-weighted image (Fig. 15B) shows the right lateral ventricle with replacement of normal cerebrospinal fluid (CSF) signal by an isointense substance that has a border of obviously increased high signal intensity. The axial T1-weighted images (Figs. 15C and D) show the presence of a serpentine high signal within the posterior right temporal lobe, as well as a high signal within the right ventricular trigone and third ventricle. Note the CSF level in the contralateral (left) trigone shown in Fig. 15C (*arrow*).

Diagnosis

Intraventricular hemorrhage (complicating previous infarction).

Discussion

Primary intraventricular hemorrhage is uncommon. It has been described with aneurysms, vascular malformations, and tumors within the choroid plexus or on the anterior choroidal or lenticular striate vessels. Pituitary tumors complicated by pituitary apoplexy, disorders, or coagulation may also predispose to such hemorrhages. In a number of reported instances, no etiology could be established. The clinical presentation is generally acute onset of headache, nausea, and vomiting together with an alteration of mental state.

In this case, it is tempting to postulate that the presence of recent occlusive disease in the distribution of the right middle cerebral artery led to an increase in hydrostatic pressure within the deep perforating vessels that remained patent and, when coupled with failure of autoregulation in the face of a blood pressure elevation, produced the intraventricular hemorrhage. The striking demonstration of magnetic susceptibility effect at this high (1.5 T) field is well demonstrated, together with the early formation of methemoglobin in the periphery of this bleed.

References

1. Gates PC, Barnett HJ, Vinters HV. Primary intraventricular hemorrhage in adults. *Stroke* 1986;17:872–876.
2. Grabe DA, Robertson WD, LaPointe JS. Computed tomographic diagnosis of intraventricular hemorrhage. *Radiology* 1982;143:91–96.
3. Gomori JM, Grossman RI, Hackney DB. Variable appearances of subacute intracranial hematomas on high field spin-echo MR. *AJNR* 1987;8:1019–1026.

Submitted by: Michael Brant-Zawadzki, M.D., Senior Editor.

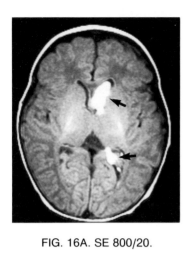

FIG. 16A. SE 800/20.

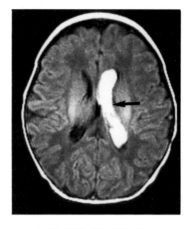

FIG. 16B. SE 800/20.

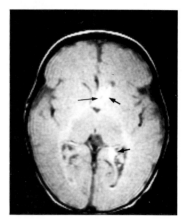

FIG. 16C. SE 2,800/30.

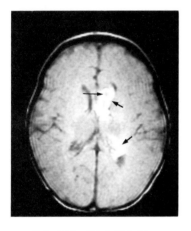

FIG. 16D. SE 2,800/30.

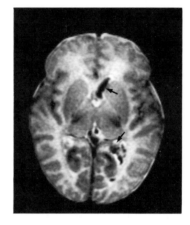

FIG. 16E. SE 2,800/90.

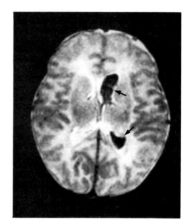

FIG. 16F. SE 2,800/90.

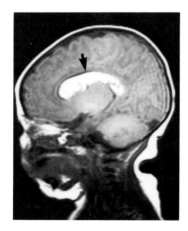

FIG. 16G. SE 800/20.

Clinical History

A 3-week-old premature infant with seizures.

Findings

Axial T2-W (SE 2,800/30 and 90), sagittal T1-W (SE 800/20), and axial T1-W (SE 800/20) images are provided for review. The axial and sagittal T1-weighted images show high signal material nearly filling the left lateral ventricle (Figs. 16A, B, and G, *arrows*). On the SE 2,800/30 axial images, the material remains mostly high signal (Figs. 16C and D, *short arrows*); however, some lower signal is now noted in the center of the material in the anterior horn (Figs. 16C and D, *long arrows*). On the SE 2,800/90 axial images, the material becomes very low signal (Figs. 16E and F, *arrows*).

Diagnosis

Early subacute hematoma in germinal matrix.

Discussion

The findings in this case are consistent with early subacute hemorrhage, representing intracellular methemoglobin, which shortens T2 and T1 (see Table 1, Case 8).

Intracerebral hemorrhage develops in 40–70% of neonates weighing less than 1,500 g. These neonatal hemorrhages originate in the germinal matrix, a loose network of highly vascular tissue with little supporting stroma that contains primitive nerve cells and is located in the ependymal lining the lateral wall of the lateral ventricle. The germinal matrix is largest in the region of the head of the caudate nucleus. The exact cause of germinal-matrix hemorrhage is uncertain, but cerebral hypoxia related to neonatal respiratory distress, which is frequently associated with cardiac and vasomotor instability, is thought to predispose to this hemorrhage. The hemorrhage usually develops during the first four days of life and is frequently not present at birth. The hemorrhages range in degree from mild to very severe. They may be localized in one or several regions of the germinal matrix. The head of the caudate nucleus adjacent to the frontal horn is the site most frequently involved. Varying degrees of intraventricular rupture occur in the majority of cases, being mild in approximately 25%. Large brain hemorrhage or ventricular hemorrhage develops in approximately 25% and carries a grave prognosis. Small intraventricular hemorrhages clear by seven to nine days, whereas large ones take up to two weeks, and parenchymal hemorrhages may take up to three months to resolve. Intraventricular hemorrhage leads to hydrocephalus in approximately one-third of cases, more commonly with larger hemorrhages.

Reference

1. Burstein J, Papile LA, Burstein R. Intraventricular hemorrhage and hydrocephalus in premature newborns: a prospective study with CT. *AJR* 1979;132:631–635.

Submitted by: Louis M. Teresi, M.D. and Stephen J. Davis, M.D., Huntington Medical Research Institutes, Pasadena, California; William G. Bradley, Jr., M.D., Ph.D., Senior Editor.

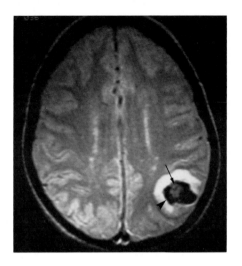

FIG. 17A. SE 2,800/30.

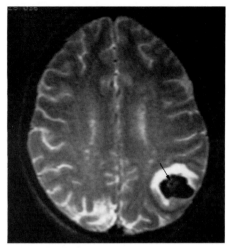

FIG. 17B. SE 2,800/70.

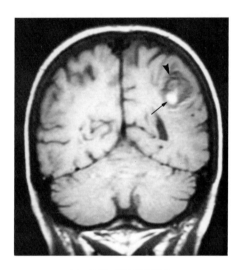

FIG. 17C. SE 800/20.

Clinical History

A 71-year-old woman with new-onset seizures.

Findings

Axial T2-W (SE 2,800/30 and 70) and sagittal T1-W (SE 800/20) images are provided for review. The axial SE 2,800/30 image shows a complex mass in the posterior left parietal lobe (Fig. 17A). The mass has a slightly hypointense center (Fig. 17A, *long arrow*), which becomes more hypointense on the SE 2,800/70 image (Fig. 17B, *long arrow*) and is hyperintense on the SE 800/20 coronal image (Fig. 17C, *long arrow*).

On the SE 2,800/30 axial image, the center of the lesion is surrounded by a markedly hypointense region (Fig. 17A, *arrowhead*), which is persistently hypointense on the SE 2,800/70 image (Fig. 17B) and isointense on the SE 800/20 coronal image (Fig. 17C, *arrowhead*).

Diagnosis

Acute and early subacute hemorrhage.

Discussion

This hemorrhage is complex. There are MR signal changes consistent with intracellular deoxyhemoglobin (Figs. 17A and C, *arrowhead*), which is hypointense on T2-weighted images but isointense on T1-weighted images. There are signal changes consistent with intracellular methemoglobin (Figs. 17A and C, *long arrow*), which is hypointense on T2-weighted images but hyperintense on T1-weighted images. The high-signal periphery of the lesion seen only on the T2-weighted images is consistent with edema. Thus, this hemorrhage shows signs of acute and early subacute hemorrhage. When staging a hemorrhage, the most advanced stage should be quoted: e.g., in this case, "early subacute" should be used to describe the hematoma.

References

1. Gomori JM, Grossman RI. Mechanisms responsible for the appearance and evolution of intracranial hemorrhage. *Radiographics* 1990;8:427–451.
2. Bradley WG. Hemorrhage. In: Bradley WG, Bydder G, eds. *MRI atlas of the brain.* New York: Raven Press/London: Martin Dunitz, 1990;205.

Submitted by: Louis M. Teresi, M.D. and Stephen J. Davis, M.D., Huntington Medical Research Institutes, Pasadena, California; William G. Bradley, Jr., M.D., Ph.D., Senior Editor.

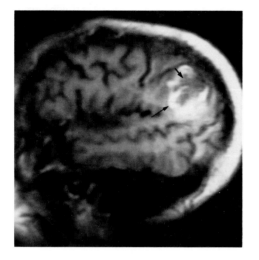

FIG. 18A. SE 800/20.

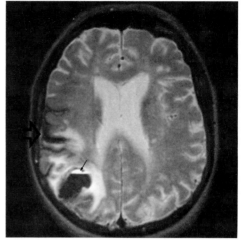

FIG. 18B. SE 2,800/70.

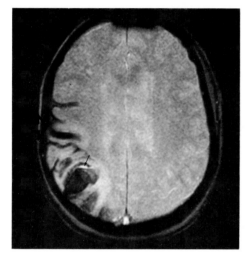

FIG. 18C. GRE 75/20/10°.

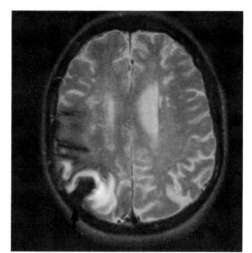

FIG. 18D. SE 2,800/70.

Clinical History

A 77-year-old woman with a history of left arm and leg numbness.

Findings

Axial T2-W (SE 2,800/70), sagittal T1-W (SE 800/20), and gradient-echo (GRE 75/20/10°) images are provided for review. The sagittal SE 800/20 image shows a mass in the right posterior parietal lobe (Fig. 18A). The mass has an isointense center (Fig. 18A, *short arrow*) and a hyperintense rim (Fig. 18A, *long arrow*). The SE 2,800/70 image shows that the lesion is almost uniformly hypointense, with a small high-signal fluid level (Fig. 18B, *small arrow*). On the gradient echo images, the mass remains hypointense, yet somewhat heterogeneous (Fig. 18C). The small fluid level remains bright (Fig. 18C, *small arrow*).

The SE 2,800/70 axial images also show diffuse low signal in cortex of the right parietal lobe (Fig. 18B, *open arrow*). This low signal becomes more pronounced on the gradient echo study (Fig. 18C, *open arrow*).

Diagnosis

Acute to early subacute hematoma with fluid level and cortical siderosis.

Discussion

Many investigators have noted that gradient-echo MR imaging can depict acute and chronic hemorrhage not seen with conventional spin-echo techniques. This heightened sensitivity of gradient-echo imaging is attributed to magnetic susceptibility-induced static-field inhomogeneities arising from the paramagnetic blood and its breakdown products, which shorten T2. The spin-echo sequence is not sensitive to static-field inhomogeneities because the echo is acquired with a 180-degree refocusing pulse, which rephases both susceptibility-induced dephasing and phase incoherence from inhomogeneities in the static applied magnetic field. In contrast, the gradient reversal used for echo formation in gradient-echo imaging rephases only what application of the gradient itself has dephased.

Superficial cortical siderosis refers to the staining of the cortex with hemosiderin following subarachnoid hemorrhage. The evolution of methemoglobin to hemosiderin in the subarachnoid space with subsequent cortical persistence may occur in the months following subarachnoid hemorrhage. Indeed, this patient's hematoma cavity communicates with the superficial cortex (Fig. 18D, *arrow*). High field and gradient-echo techniques are the most sensitive for detecting the parenchymal hemosiderin because of their sensitivity to the magnetic susceptibility properties of hemosiderin.

References

1. Atlas SW, Mark AS, Grossman RI, et al. Intracranial hemorrhage: gradient-echo MR imaging at 1.5 T. Comparison with spin-echo imaging and clinical applications. *AJNR* 1989;10:656.
2. Gomori J, Grossman R, Golbert H, et al. High-field MR imaging of superficial siderosis of the central nervous system. *J Comput Assist Tomogr* 1985;9:972–975.

Submitted by: Louis M. Teresi, M.D. and Stephen J. Davis, M.D., Huntington Medical Research Institutes, Pasadena, California; William G. Bradley, Jr., M.D., Ph.D., Senior Editor.

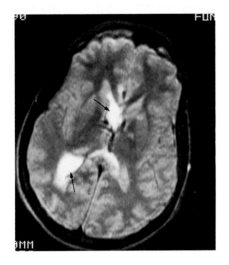
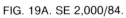
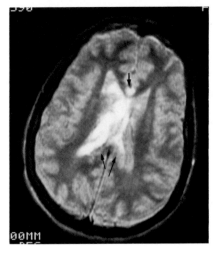
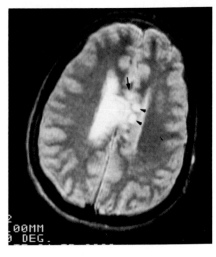

FIG. 19A. SE 2,000/84.　　　FIG. 19B. SE 2,000/84.　　　FIG. 19C. SE 2,000/84.

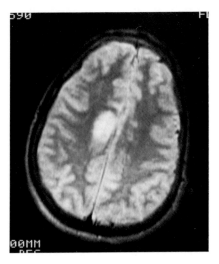
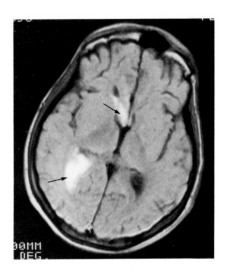

FIG. 19D. SE 2,000/84.　　　FIG. 19E. SE 778/28.

46

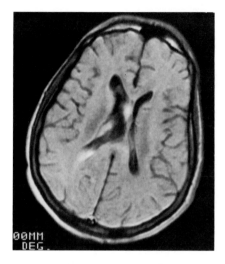
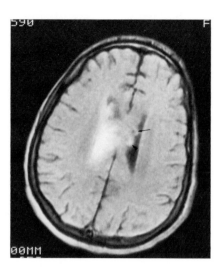
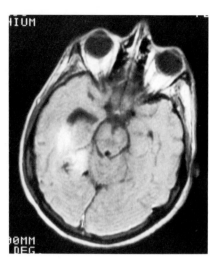

FIG. 19F. SE 778/28.   FIG. 19G. SE 778/28.   FIG. 19H. SE 778/28 with Gd-DTPA.

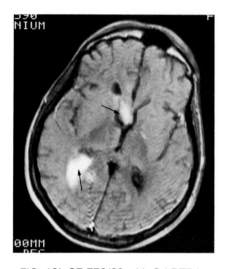
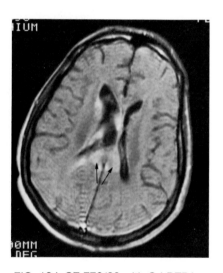

FIG. 19I. SE 778/28 with Gd-DTPA.   FIG. 19J. SE 778/28 with Gd-DTPA.

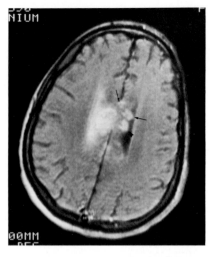

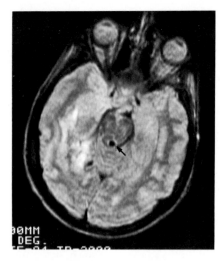

FIG. 19K. SE 778/28 with Gd-DTPA.

FIG. 19L. SE 2,000/84.

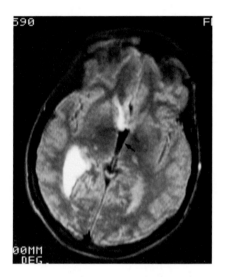

FIG. 19M. SE 2,000/84.

Clinical History

A 26-year-old man who was found unconscious after a high-velocity motor vehicle accident.

48

Findings

Axial T2-W (SE 2,000/84) and axial T1-W (SE 778/28) images before and after intravenous gadolinium-DTPA administration are provided for review. The axial SE 2,000/84 images show high-intensity material in the frontal and occipital horns of the right lateral ventricle (Fig. 19A, *arrows*). A hyperintense focus is seen in the genu of the corpus callosum (Fig. 19B, *short arrow*). Subtle increased signal intensity is also seen in the splenium of the corpus callosum (Fig. 19C, *arrow*). Two foci of increased signal are seen in the body of the corpus callosum (Fig. 19C, *arrowheads*).

The SE 778/28 axial images show that the material in the ventricle is hyperintense (Fig. 19E, *arrows*). The focus of increased signal intensity in the genu of the corpus callosum is not seen on the SE 778/28 image (Fig. 19F). The more anterior of the two foci of increased signal intensity in the body of the corpus callosum is slightly hypointense on the SE 778/28 image (Fig. 19G, *long arrow*) and the more posterior is hyperintense (Fig. 19G, *arrowhead*).

After gadolinium administration, the foci in the genu and body of the corpus callosum attain a higher signal intensity (Fig. 19K, *arrows/arrowhead*). The splenium of the corpus callosum also enhances slightly (Fig. 19J, *arrows*).

The ventricles are enlarged out of proportion to the cortical sulci for this 26-year-old. There is particularly noticeable enlargement of the third ventricle (Fig. 19M, *arrow*) and aqueduct (Fig. 19L, *arrow*). Marked flow void is noted in the aqueduct, extending into the dilated third ventricle.

Diagnosis

Shear injury of corpus callosum (with and without hemorrhage), late subacute intraventricular hemorrhage, and communicating hydrocephalus.

Discussion

Impact injury deforms different loci of the brain substance to different degrees, and internal shearing and stress can traumatize even deep-lying cells and their processes. Diffuse axon and neuron cell body injury may be scattered throughout. Shearing injuries result when asymmetric pressure is exerted on the white matter and deep gray matter. Such shearing injuries result in local hemorrhage or edema in both white and deep gray matter. This is the result of the brain moving in a sagittal plane or rotating in the skull around the axis of the brainstem. The most common locations for shearing injuries are the subcortical gray-white matter interfaces, internal capsule, pons and midbrain, and corpus callosum. The vast majority of diffuse axonal injuries involving the corpus callosum involve the splenium. Shearing injuries involving the corpus callosum indicate a poor outcome, with most ending up in a persistent vegetative state or death. Approximately 35% of patients with hemorrhagic shear injuries of the corpus callosum have intraventricular hemorrhage.

In a series of 40 patients, diffuse axonal injury comprised 48.2% of all traumatic lesions (1). When present, they tended to be multiple, with 50.3% of the lesions found in the 15 patients with the most severe initial impairment of consciousness. Although most of the lesions were nonhemorrhagic, 18% contained small foci of blood. Hemorrhage within diffuse axonal lesions occurred more often in those portions of the white matter with the most vascularity, the subcortical regions. The size of the diffuse axonal lesions ranged from 5 to 15 mm and varied in location. Peripheral lesions tended to be smaller than central ones.

In this case, enhancement of the lesions in the corpus callosum is consistent with blood-brain barrier breakdown associated with shear-type injury. This is seen in both hemorrhagic and nonhemorrhagic lesions.

Reference

1. Gentry LR, Godersky JC, Thompson B. MR imaging of head trauma: review of the distribution and radiopathic features of traumatic lesions. *AJNR* 1988;9:101–110.

Submitted by: Louis M. Teresi, M.D. and Stephen J. Davis, M.D., Huntington Medical Research Institutes, Pasadena, California; William G. Bradley, Jr., M.D., Ph.D., Senior Editor.

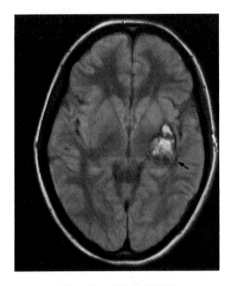

FIG. 20A. SE 2,000/30.

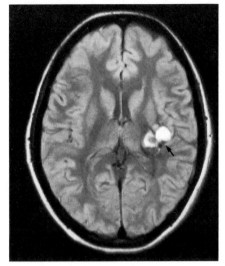

FIG. 20B. SE 2,000/30.

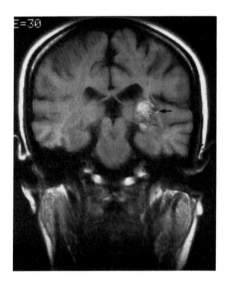

FIG. 20C. SE 500/30.

Clinical History

A 33-year-old woman with fibromuscular dysplasia.

Findings

Axial proton density-weighted (SE 2,000/30) and coronal T1-W (SE 500/30) images are provided for review. The SE 2,000/30 axial images show a mass of mixed signal intensity in the posterior basal ganglia on the left (Figs. 20A and B, *arrows*). Regions of the mass are very hyperintense, whereas others are very hypointense. The coronal SE 500/30 image shows similar changes (Fig. 20C, *arrow*).

Diagnosis

Chronic basal ganglia hemorrhage.

Discussion

The findings in this case are consistent with chronic hemorrhage. The chronic stage begins after approximately two weeks and represents lysed red blood cells and blood breakdown products. The whole hematoma appears hyperintense on all image pulse sequences due to free methemoglobin, which may persist for months and perhaps years. Reactive macrophages that accumulate on the hematoma periphery digest the hemoglobin products and deposit insoluble hemosiderin granules in their lysosomes. These hemosiderin-laden macrophages are not removed from the brain and persist indefinitely in the hematoma periphery. After approximately two weeks in the cerebral parenchyma immediately adjacent to the hematoma, there appears a ring of marked hypointensity on T2-weighted images, particularly at high field, which is mildly hypointense on T1-weighted images, corresponding to hemosiderin-laden macrophages.

Hypertensive hemorrhage occurs in the putamen, thalamus, cerebellum, pons, and, less commonly, at other sites, usually in the lobar white matter. Such hemorrhages are caused by rupture of microaneurysms situated on the small perforating arteries arising from the circle of Willis. The putamen is the most common site, accounting for at least 50% of hypertensive hemorrhages. The thalamus is the second most common site. Hemorrhages at these two sites are distinct clinically except when massive and both sites are involved. Intraventricular extension from these sites is common. Cerebellar hemorrhages, usually in the dentate nucleus, are associated with a high mortality. Of hypertensive hemorrhages, 9% are in the pons, starting centrally and usually extending superiorly to the midbrain. When there is no history of hypertension, arteriography may be helpful in the diagnosis of arteriovenous malformation, aneurysm, or neoplasm associated with hemorrhage.

Reference

1. Walshe TM, Hier DB, Davis KR. The diagnosis of hypertensive intracerebral hemorrhage: the contribution of CT. *Comput Tomogr* 1977;1:63–69.

Submitted by: Louis M. Teresi, M.D. and Stephen J. Davis, M.D., Huntington Medical Research Institutes, Pasadena, California; William G. Bradley, Jr., M.D., Ph.D., Senior Editor.

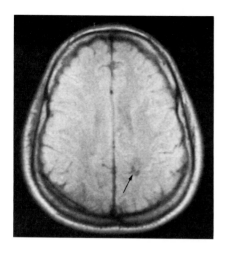

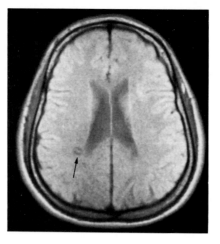

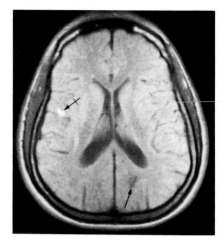

FIG. 21A. SE 2,100/30.

FIG. 21B. SE 2,100/30.

FIG. 21C. SE 2,100/30.

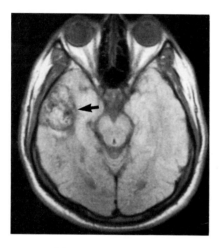

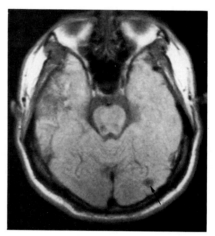

FIG. 21D. SE 2,100/30.

FIG. 21E. SE 2,100/30.

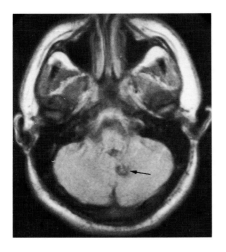 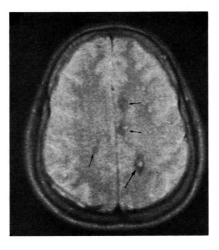 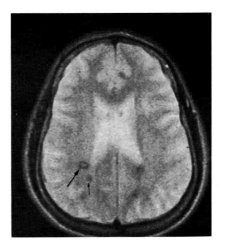

FIG. 21F. SE 2,100/30.   FIG. 21G. SE 2,100/100.   FIG. 21H. SE 2,100/100.

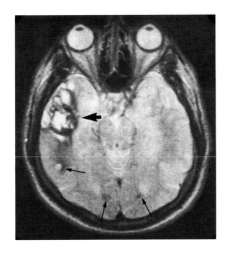 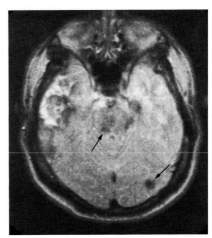

FIG. 21I. SE 2,100/100.   FIG. 21J. SE 2,100/100.

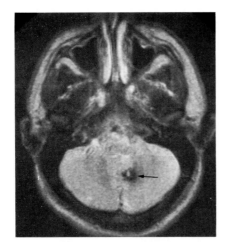

FIG. 21K. SE 2,100/100.

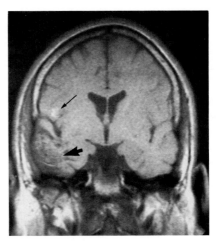

FIG. 21L. SE 700/26.

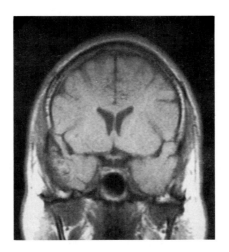

FIG. 21M. SE 700/26.

Clinical History

A 34-year-old man with skin lesions and a family history of bleeding disorders.

Findings

Axial T2-W (SE 2,100/30 and 100) and coronal T1-W (SE 700/26) images are provided for review. The axial SE 2,100/30 images show multiple small, low-signal foci scattered throughout the subcortical and deep white matter of the supratentorial and infratentorial compartments (Figs. 21A–E, *small arrows*). A small high-signal focus is seen in the right temporal lobe (Fig. 21C, *crossed arrow*). A large complex mass is also seen in the anterior right temporal lobe. The mass is essentially isointense but has a low-signal periphery, with multiple low-signal internal components. On the SE 2,100/100 sequence, the low-signal periphery of the mass becomes much more prominent, as do some of the low-signal internal components (Fig. 21I, *arrow*). Other areas of the mass become very high signal. The SE 2,100/100 images also show that the multiple foci of low signal intensity become larger and lower signal on the SE 2,100/100 compared with the SE 2,100/30 images (Figs. 21G–K, *small arrows*). The coronal SE 700/26 images show that the large complex mass in the right temporal lobe is an isointense structure (Fig. 21L, *large arrow*). The very prominent low-signal periphery and internal components are not seen on this sequence. A small focus of increased signal is seen in the right parietal lobe (Fig. 21L, *small arrow*), corresponding to the high-signal focus on the SE 2,100/30 and 100 sequences.

Diagnosis

Encephalomalacia with siderosis right temporal lobe, multiple foci of chronic hemorrhage, consistent with multiple telangietasias, and single focus of late-subacute hemorrhage.

Discussion

As stated previously, hemosiderin-laden macrophages are not removed from the brain and persist indefinitely in the hematoma periphery. After approximately two weeks, a peripheral ring appears of marked hypointensity on T2-weighted images with long inter-echo interval at high field, which is mildly hypointense on T1-weighted and proton density-weighted images, corresponding to hemosiderin-laden macrophages. This is due to the superparamagnetic properties of hemosiderin: its T2 relaxation rate increases quadratically with field strength and increases with lengthening of the spin-echo interecho interval and TE.

Superficial cortical siderosis refers to the staining of the cortex with hemosiderin following subarachnoid hemorrhage; however, it is also noted in encephalomalacia from resorbed hematomas. High-field and gradient-echo techniques are the most sensitive for detecting the parenchymal hemosiderin because of their sensitivity to the magnetic susceptibility properties of hemosiderin.

Multiple telangiectasias are part of Osler-Weber-Rendu disease with telangiectasias of the skin, and of the mucosa of the oropharynx with pulmonary arteriovenous malformations (AVMs) and visceral telangiectasias. The lesions can be seen in children; however, the appearance of these lesions increases with age, peaking in the fourth and fifth decades of life. This correlates with the frequency and severity of hemorrhagic episodes. It is transmitted as an autosomal dominant trait. Thus, a family history of bleeding in both sexes is verifiable. The telangiectasias result from dilation and convolution of venules and capillaries. Vessel walls are thinned to the level of a single layer of endothelium that has neither anatomic support nor contractile properties. These fragile, angiomatous masses of vascular components bleed spontaneously or following minor trauma. Telangiectasias are difficult to diagnose with angiography. A small blush with normal arteries and veins is rarely seen. More often they bleed, and the diagnosis made on CT or MR is intracerebral hemorrhage.

Pulmonary arteriovenous fistulas may be responsible for septic cerebral emboli. True AVMs of the cerebral, hepatic, and splenic circulations can be associated with diffuse multiple telangiectasias.

References

1. Gomori JM, Grossman RI. Mechanisms responsible for the appearance and evolution of intracranial hemorrhage. *Radiographics* 1988;8:427–451.
2. Gomori J, Grossman R, Golbert H, et al. High-field MR imaging of superficial siderosis of the central nervous system. *J Comput Assist Tomogr* 1985;9:972–975.
3. Nathan DG. Hematologic diseases. In: Wyngaarden JB, Smith LH, eds. *Cecil: textbook of medicine.* Philadelphia: WB Saunders, 1988;1060.

Submitted by: Louis M. Teresi, M.D., Stephen J. Davis, M.D., and Mark Ziemba, M.D., Huntington Medical Research Institutes, Pasadena, California; William G. Bradley, Jr., M.D., Ph.D., Senior Editor.

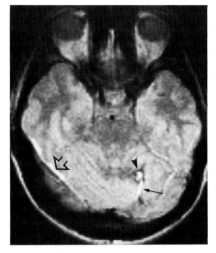

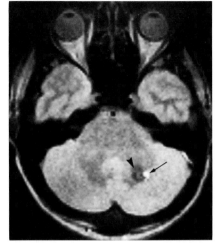

FIG. 22A. SE 2,000/56.   FIG. 22B. SE 2,000/56.

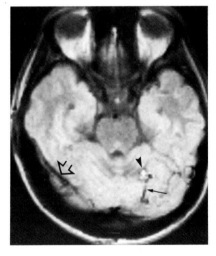

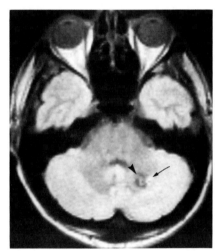

FIG. 22C. SE 2,000/28.   FIG. 22D. SE 2,000/28.

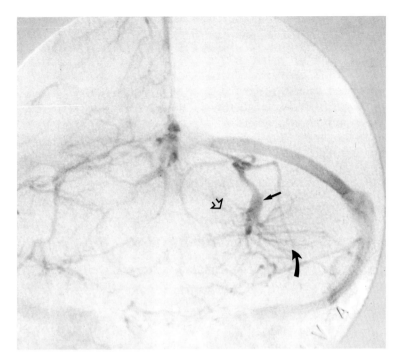

FIG. 22E. Angiogram.

Clinical History

A 36-year-old man with a long history of seizures.

Findings

Axial T2-W (SE 2,000/28 and 56) images and venous-phase cerebral angiogram are provided for review. The SE 2,000/56 image shows a high-signal linear structure extending through the left cerebellar hemisphere (Fig. 22A, *arrow*). A high-signal focus with a low-signal halo is associated with it in the deep cerebellar white matter (Fig. 22A, *arrowhead*). On the SE 2,000/28 image, the high-signal linear structure now appears as a signal void (Fig. 22C, *arrow*). Of note are similar signal changes in the right sigmoid sinus (Figs. 22A and C, *open arrows*). The low-signal halo around the high-signal focus is less prominent (Fig. 22C, *arrowhead*). The SE 2,000/56 image shows a low-signal focus (Fig. 22B, *arrowhead*) associated with a very high-signal focus (Fig. 22B, *arrow*). Both low- and high-signal foci are less prominent on the SE 2,000/28 study (Fig. 22D).

The venous phase of a cerebral angiogram shows a prominent vein (Fig. 22E, *straight arrow*) draining into the superior cerebellar vein, with numerous tributary veins feeding into it (Fig. 22E, *curved arrow*). On the medial side of the vein, the small tributary branches are indistinct and distorted (Fig. 22E, *open arrow*), corresponding to the region of suspected hemorrhage on the MR images.

Diagnosis

Venous angioma showing even-echo rephasing, associated with chronic hemorrhage.

Discussion

Venous angiomas are composed solely of veins. The abnormality consists of either an enlarged single vein with many tributaries or a compact group of such veins. They represent the rarest form of vascular malformation. They occur in both the cerebrum and cerebellum, but the most frequent site is the spinal cord and meninges. They are often asymptomatic but may be associated with subarachnoid and intracerebral hemorrhage or with seizures. If thrombosis occurs in the draining vein, hemorrhage might occur (as is frequently seen with venous thrombosis in the brain). Spontaneous hemorrhage otherwise does not occur unless there is an increase in intracranial pressure. Cerebellar venous angiomas are more prone to bleed spontaneously. Angiograms show a normal arterial and capillary phase, with multiple venules draining in an umbrella-like pattern toward an engorged draining vein, which is often positioned perpendicular to the cortex.

Review of Flow Enhancement Phenomena in MR Imaging. Three causes of signal loss have been described due to flow. These are high velocity signal loss (or time-of-flight loss), turbulence, and first echo dephasing. High velocity signal loss results from protons moving through the selected slice too rapidly to be excited by both the 90° RF pulse and the 180° RF pulse needed to produce a spin echo. Turbulence produces irreversible dephasing due to random motion of fluid elements. First echo dephasing results from protons in the voxel having different velocities and, therefore, different rates of phase accumulation as they flow into a magnetic field gradient. The resultant dephasing produces reversible signal loss which can be reconstituted if a symmetric second echo image is acquired (see even echo rephasing below). Three causes of increased signal intensity due to motion have been described for MR imaging: diastolic pseudogating, flow-related enhancement (FRE) or entry phenomenon, and even-echo rephasing.

Stagnant, unclotted blood has a fairly high signal intensity on T2-weighted MR images due to the relatively long T2 relaxation time. Thus, when there is marked slowing of flow or vascular obstruction, the signal from blood is increased. When there is apparent slowing of arterial flow due to "diastolic pseudogating," intraluminal signal is also increased. Diastolic pseudogating results from chance synchronization of the cardiac and MR cycles. This can occur, for example, if the heart rate is 60 (one cardiac cycle per second) and the TR of the imager is set to one second. Should the two cycles then remain in phase for a four-minute acquisition, several slices would be acquired during diastole and several during systole. Those sections acquired during the slow-flow diastole would demonstrate higher intraluminal signal than those acquired during high-flow systole. Whenever high intraluminal signal is seen in an artery, diastolic pseudogating should be excluded as an etiology by acquiring images at the same level, gating to cardiac systole.

When totally magnetized (unsaturated) protons flow into the entry slice of a multi-slice imaging volume, high intraluminal signal can result. Optimally, the flow rate should be such that all of the blood within the slice is replaced during one repetition time. For slices approximately 1 cm thick and TR on the order of one second, this corresponds to velocities on the order of 1 cm/sec.

This phenomenon has been called "flow-related enhancement" or "entry phenomenon." It is most prominent near the entry surface for the in-flowing blood and for slow flow rates (venous). As the flow rate increases, FRE can be observed, but the signal-decreasing dephasing and time-of-flight effects result in counteracting signal loss. Flow-related enhancement is increased on short TR, T1-weighted images. Although the intraluminal signal does not increase, the shorter TR allows less time for recovery of the adjacent stationary tissues; thus, the relative signal intensity within the blood vessel is higher. FRE is also increased at higher fields at a given TR due to the increase in T1 with field strength.

When dual-echo sequences are used and the TE of the second echo is exactly twice that of the first, the phenomenon of "even-echo rephasing" can occur. This is only seen in slow laminar flow (e.g., veins and dural sinuses).

The signal loss observed on the first echo due to dephasing can be entirely reconstituted if the velocity is constant until the second echo. While even-echo rephasing is most often observed in veins, it can also be seen in flowing cerebrospinal fluid and should be considered when high signal is observed within the basal cisterns or ventricular system, particularly on an entry slice.

Rephasing can be operator-induced by using rephasing gradients that force the phase of constant-velocity moving spins to be zero at the echo. This is observed when extra gradient pulses are applied to suppress motion artifact, a technique known as "gradient moment nulling." In this technique, opposing gradients are applied that eliminate any phase incoherence induced by motion (4). The effect on slowly flowing blood may be complete rephasing and, therefore, increased signal.

References

1. Rothfus GH, Albright AL, Casey KF, et al. Cerebellar venous angioma: "benign" entity? *AJNR* 1984;5:61–66.
2. Toro VE, Geyer CA, Sherman JL, et al. Cerebral venous angioma: MR findings. *AJNR* 1989;10:1133.
3. Bradley WG. Flow phenomenon. In: Stark DD, Bradley WG, eds. *Magnetic resonance imaging.* St. Louis: CV Mosby, 1988.
4. Pattanay PM, Phillips JJ, Chiu LC, et al. Motion artifact suppression technique (MAST) for MRI imaging. *J Comput Assist Tomogr* 1987;11:196–201.

Submitted by: Louis M. Teresi, M.D., Stephen J. Davis, M.D., and Mark Ziemba, M.D., Huntington Medical Research Institutes, Pasadena, California; William G. Bradley, Jr., M.D., Ph.D., Senior Editor.

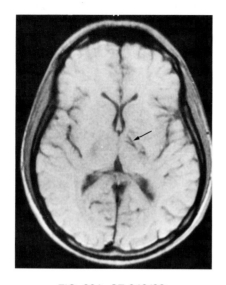

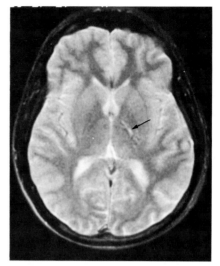

FIG. 23A. SE 649/22.   FIG. 23B. SE 3,000/85.

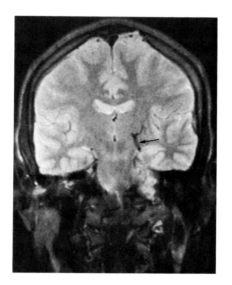

FIG. 23C. SE 2,000/85.

Clinical History

A 25-year-old man with headache.

Findings

Axial (SE 3,000/85) and coronal T2-W (SE 2,000/85) and axial T1-W (SE 649/22) images are provided for review. The axial T1-weighted image shows a low-signal linear structure in the left internal capsule (Fig. 23A, *arrow*). The axial SE 3,000/85 image shows that the low-signal linear structure assumes a high intensity (Fig. 23B, *arrow*). The coronal SE 2,000/85 image, however, shows the structure as low signal (Fig. 23C, *arrow*). Of note is the fact that the axial T2-weighted images used gradient moment-nulling motion artifact suppression, whereas the T2-weighted coronal images did not.

Diagnosis

Venous angioma evidencing induced increased signal secondary to gradient moment nulling.

Discussion

Rephasing can be artifactually induced by using rephasing gradients that force the phase of constant-velocity moving spins to be zero at the time of the echo. This is observed when extra gradient pulses are applied to suppress motion artifact, a technique known as "gradient moment nulling." In this technique, opposing gradients are applied that eliminate any phase incoherence induced by motion (2). The effect on slowly flowing blood may be to cause complete rephasing and, therefore, increased signal. It is important in evaluating flow effects on MR images to be aware of techniques used to suppress unwanted motion artifacts.

References

1. Bradley WG. Flow phenomenon. In: Stark DD, Bradley WG, eds. *Magnetic resonance imaging.* St. Louis: CV Mosby, 1988.
2. Pattanay PM, Phillips JJ, Chiu LC, et al. Motion artifact suppression technique (MAST) for MRI imaging. *J Comput Assist Tomogr* 1987;11:196–201.

Submitted by: Louis M. Teresi, M.D., Stephen J. Davis, M.D., and Mark Ziemba, M.D., Huntington Medical Research Institutes, Pasadena, California; William G. Bradley, Jr., M.D., Ph.D., Senior Editor.

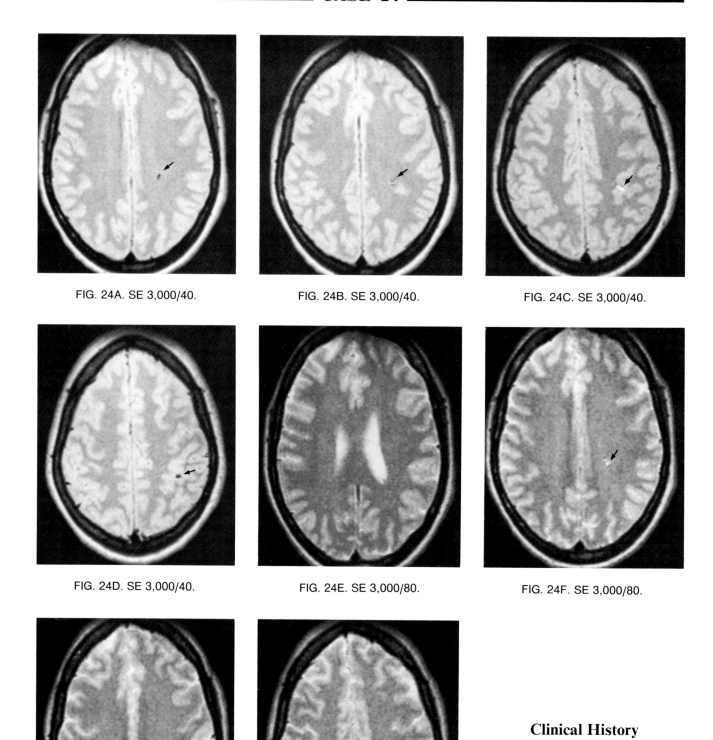

FIG. 24A. SE 3,000/40.

FIG. 24B. SE 3,000/40.

FIG. 24C. SE 3,000/40.

FIG. 24D. SE 3,000/40.

FIG. 24E. SE 3,000/80.

FIG. 24F. SE 3,000/80.

FIG. 24G. SE 3,000/80.

FIG. 24H. SE 3,000/80.

Clinical History

A 38-year-old woman with seizures.

Findings

Axial images show a low-signal circular structure within the left centrum semiovale extending from the atrium of the left lateral ventricle through the white matter of the centrum semiovale to the cortex of the parietal lobe (Figs. 24A–D, F, G, *arrows*). On Figs. 24B, C, and F–H, this tubular structure has high signal, possibly due to flow-related enhancement.

Diagnosis

Venous angioma.

Discussion

Venous angiomas are a type of vascular malformation. They are entirely venous in structure and represent the local dysplasia of medullary veins and adjacent brain. Generally, they drain into an aberrant central transparenchymal vein that subsequently empties directly into a venous sinus. Rarely, they may drain into deep vascular structures such as the thalamostriate vein. They occasionally bleed, but are more commonly associated with headaches or seizures. On MR scans, they appear as tubular structures, generally showing signal void; however, they may also show flow-related enhancement or even-echo rephasing or symmetric second-echo images.

Venous angiomas are most often clinically asymptomatic, although they may be associated with subarachnoid or intracerebral hemorrhage or with seizures. Cerebellar venous angiomas are more prone to bleed, resulting in spontaneous and often recurrent hemorrhage. In the majority of cases, a non-contrast CT scan may appear normal, although sometimes a rounded hyperdense area is seen. The contrast-enhanced CT scan shows a rounded or linear area of enhancement not associated with mass effect or surrounding edema. On MR, venous angiomas can be diagnosed without the need for intravenous contrast. The vein is generally hypointense on the first echo image, with increasing signal intensity on the second echo image; this is due to even-echo rephasing, indicating slow laminar flow. These angiomas are not usually associated with mass effect. Occasionally, prior hemorrhage may result in areas of encephalomalacia, calcification, or hemosiderin deposition.

Reference

1. Wendling LR, Moore JS, Kieffer SA, et al. Intracerebral venous angioma, *Radiology* 1976;119:141–147.

Submitted by: Louis M. Teresi, M.D., Stephen J. Davis, M.D., and Mark Ziemba, M.D., Huntington Medical Research Institutes, Pasadena, California; William G. Bradley, Jr., M.D., Ph.D., Senior Editor.

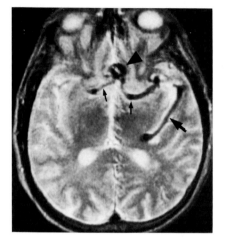

FIG. 25A. SE 3,000/85.

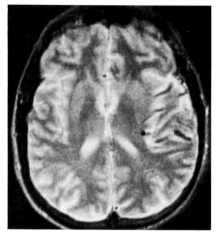

FIG. 25B. SE 3,000/85.

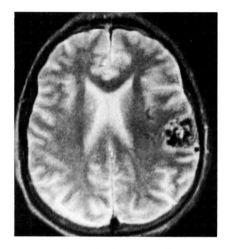

FIG. 25C. SE 3,000/85.

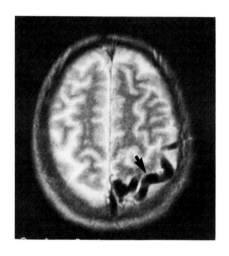

FIG. 25D. SE 3,000/85.

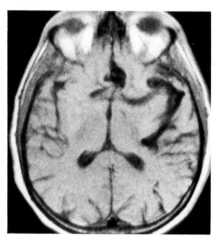

FIG. 25E. SE 649/22.

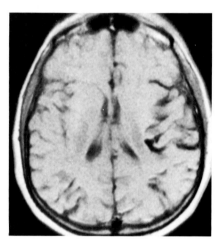

FIG. 25F. SE 649/22.

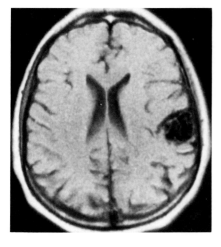

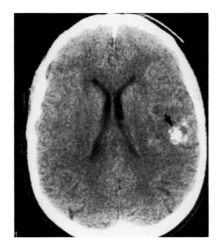

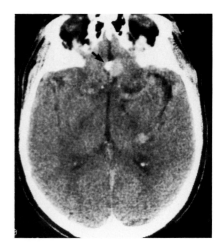

FIG. 25G. SE 649/22.   FIG. 25H. CT.   FIG. 25I. CT.

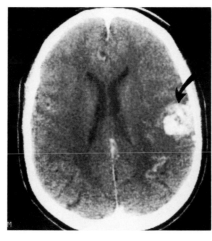

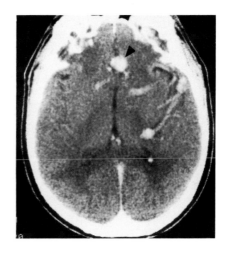

FIG. 25J. CT.   FIG. 25K. CT.

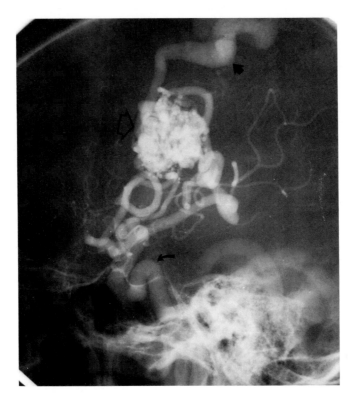

FIG. 25L. Angiogram.

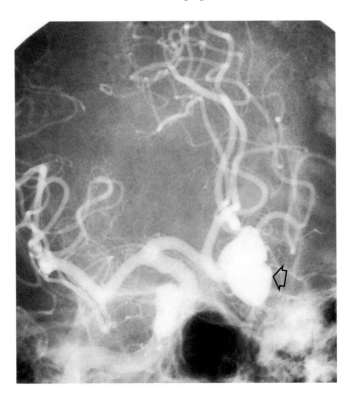

FIG. 25M. Angiogram.

Clinical History

A 56-year-old man with a history of seizures.

Findings

Axial T2-W (SE 3,000/85) and axial T1-W (SE 649/22) images are provided for review. Figure 25A (*arrowhead*) shows a rounded low-signal region in the anterior cranial fossa that does not significantly change signal intensity on the T1-weighted image (Fig. 25E). It is in the region of the anterior communicating artery, as the origins of both middle cerebral arteries can be seen (Fig. 25A, *small arrows*). The left middle cerebral artery is dilated relative to the right. A tubular-shaped low-signal structure is seen in the left insula (Fig. 25A, *large arrow*). Figure 25C shows an approximately 3 cm mass in the low left parietal lobe with mixed high and low signal intensity, remaining low signal on the T1-weighted image (Fig. 25G). The high-signal material in the center of the left parietal mass on the T2-weighted image becomes noticeably low signal on the T1-weighted image. A serpiginous low-signal structure extends over the left parietal and occipital lobes (Fig. 25D, *arrow*).

Computed tomography scans without contrast show amorphous calcifications in the right lateral portion of the rounded lesion in the anterior cranial fossa (Fig. 25I, *arrow*). With intravenous contrast, the rounded lesion enhances homogeneously (Fig. 25K, *arrowhead*). Similarly, the lesion in the left parietal lobe has numerous amorphous calcifications (Fig. 25H, *arrow*); however, it enhances inhomogenously (Fig. 25J, *curved arrow*).

The lateral view of the left internal carotid artery angiogram shows a large collection of abnormal vessels (Fig. 25L, *open arrow*), with a markedly dilated left middle cerebral artery (*curved arrows*) and draining superficial cortical vein (*short arrow*). The left posterior oblique right internal carotid artery angiogram shows the opacified lumen of a large anterior communicating artery aneurysm (Fig. 25M, *open arrow*).

Diagnosis

Parietal arteriovenous malformation, and anterior communicating artery aneurysm.

Discussion

Arteriovenous malformations (AVMs) are the most common vascular malformations of the brain. They consist of vascular clusters that form direct arteriovenous shunts without any intermediary capillary network. The afferent arteries and efferent veins are dilated and sinuous. The vessels that make up the malformations are highly variable in number, length, and caliber. Microscopically, they are between arteries and veins and often exhibit secondary changes such as thrombosis, calcification, hyalinosis, and fibrosis. The angiographic appearance is that of abnormally dilated and tortuous feeding arteries and a racemose tangle of increased vascularity, which drains early into tortuous and elongated veins. Occasionally, the malformation may become partially or completely thrombosed, and angiography may fail to show any evidence of it. The interstitial tissue is either nervous parenchyma or leptomeninges. There is often reactive gliosis at the periphery of the malformation, which is an ideal cleavage plane for the surgeon.

Three to nine percent of patients with AVMs have aneurysms. In these instances, the symptoms of the AVM (seizure and hemorrhage) usually precede those of the aneurysm. Conversely, only 0.1% of patients with aneurysms have AVMs.

Reference

1. Lee BCD, Herzberg L, Zimmerman RD, et al. MR imaging of cerebral vascular malformations. *AJNR* 1986;6:863.

Submitted by: Louis M. Teresi, M.D., Stephen J. Davis, M.D., and Mark Ziemba, M.D., Huntington Medical Research Institutes, Pasadena, California; William G. Bradley, Jr., M.D., Ph.D., Senior Editor.

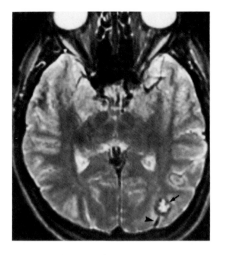

FIG. 26A. SE 2,600/100

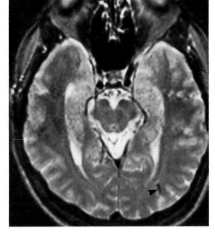

FIG. 26B. SE 2,600/100

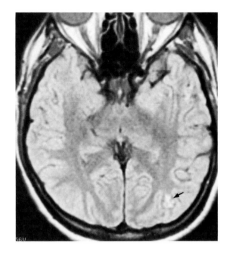

FIG. 26C. SE 2,600/25.

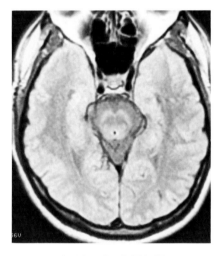

FIG. 26D. SE 2,600/25.

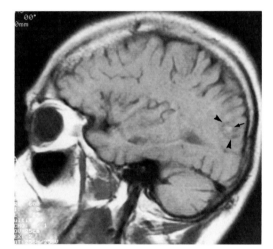

FIG. 26E. SE 600/25.

Clinical History

A 42-year-old man with new-onset seizure.

Findings

T2-weighted coronal images (Figs. 32A and B) reveal two lesions, both showing preferential low signal intensity, particularly in their periphery, fading into the nearby brain. Note the lack of surrounding edema or mass effect. Also, some high-signal internal components can be discerned. The gradient-echo image (Fig. 32C) of the left temporal lesion (the right parietal showed similar characteristics) corroborates the magnetic-susceptibility effect. In addition, no obvious feeding vessels are present (note the high signal in normal vascular structures elsewhere within the brain, particularly the basilar artery). The T1-weighted image (Fig. 32D) reveals that the left temporal lesion contains internal high signal within the low-signal border (the right parietal lesion showed similar characteristics).

Diagnosis

Multiple cavernous angiomas (occult arteriovenous malformations).

Discussion

The cavernous arteriovenous malformation or angioma is a characteristic brain parenchymal lesion on histology, as it contains almost no intervening brain parenchyma among the abnormally enlarged, thin-walled vascular channels. It can vary from a small petechial lesion of a few millimeters to a larger, well-circumscribed "mulberry-like" hemorrhagic mass many centimeters in size. The majority are single lesions, but multiple lesions may represent more than 25% of the cases studied at autopsy. Multiple lesions are now becoming recognized, due to the high sensitivity of MRI to blood by-products. A familial incidence of multiple cavernous angiomas has been described.

The hallmark of the diagnosis is the recognition of hemorrhage in various stages of development, as in this case, where the peripheral hemosiderin deposition and the internal high signal from more recent methemoglobin component is seen. Typically, there is lack of mass effect and edema: calcification will be shown on CT scans with minimal, if any, enhancement. No large feeding vessels are observed.

Finally, although the appearance of these lesions is quite specific, occasionally, hemorrhagic metastatic foci could simulate such a picture. Therefore, if any doubt exists, follow-up scan is mandatory. Clues to the presence of underlying malignancy include presence of surrounding edema, mass effect, and (of course) known primary tumor elsewhere.

References

1. Rigamonti D, Drayer BP, Johnson PC. The MRI appearance of cavernous malformations (angiomas). *J Neurosurg* 1987;67:518–524.
2. Rutka JT, Brant-Zawadzki M, Wilson CB, et al. Familial cavernous malformations: diagnostic potential of magnetic resonance imaging. *Surg Neurol* 1988;29:467–474.
3. Sze G, Krol G, Olsen WL, et al. Hemorrhagic neoplasms: MR mimic of occult vascular malformations. *Am J Radiol* 1987;149:1223–1230.

Submitted by: Michael Brant-Zawadzki, M.D., Senior Editor.

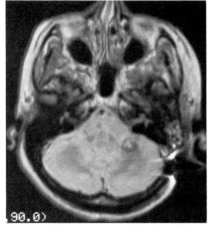

FIG. 33A. SE 3,000/30.

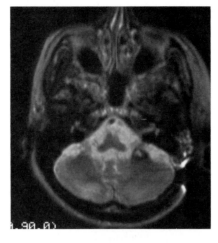

FIG. 33B. SE 3,000/75.

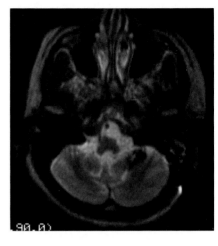

FIG. 33C. SE 3,000/75.

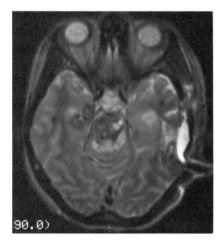

FIG. 33D. SE 3,000/75.

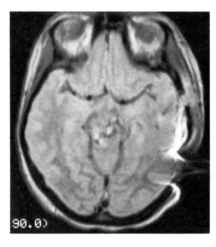

FIG. 33E. SE 3,000/30.

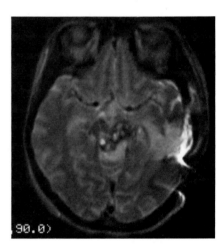

FIG. 33F. SE 3,000/75.

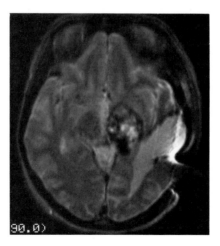

FIG. 33G. SE 3,000/75.

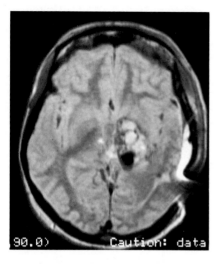

FIG. 33H. SE 3,000/30.

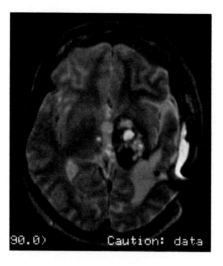

FIG. 33I. SE 3,000/75.

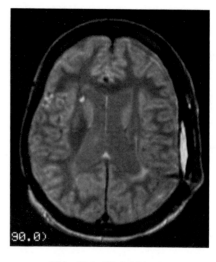

FIG. 33J. SE 3,000/30.

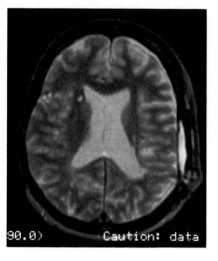

FIG. 33K. SE 3,000/75.

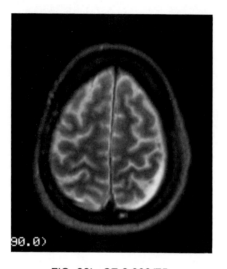

FIG. 33L. SE 3,000/75.

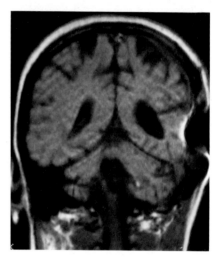

FIG. 33M. SE 700/20.

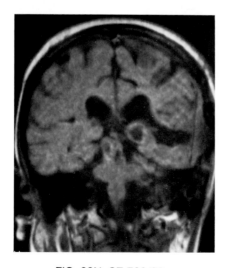

FIG. 33N. SE 700/20.

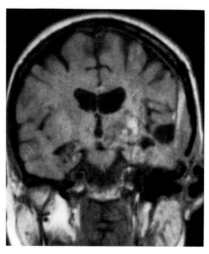

FIG. 33O. SE 700/20.

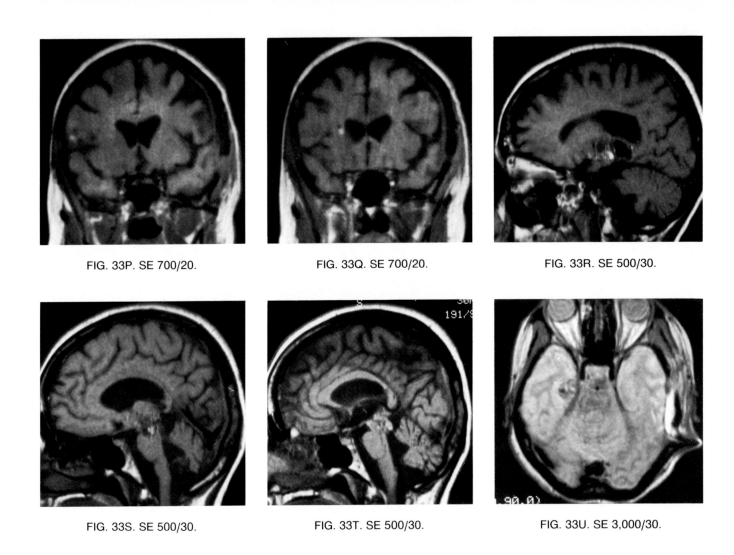

FIG. 33P. SE 700/20.　　　　FIG. 33Q. SE 700/20.　　　　FIG. 33R. SE 500/30.

FIG. 33S. SE 500/30.　　　　FIG. 33T. SE 500/30.　　　　FIG. 33U. SE 3,000/30.

Clinical History

A 38-year-old woman with a history of multiple cerebral hemorrhagic events since the age of 2 years; chronic seizure disorder with a spastic quadriparesis, speech deficit, and visual disorder. There has been previous surgery and radiation therapy.

Findings

There are multiple focal parenchymal brain abnormalities. A 4 cm complex mass involves the left basal ganglia, internal capsule, and thalamus and extends to involve the midbrain and upper pons (Figs. 33D–I, O, and R–T). This lesion may be continuous with a 2 cm lesion involving the uncus of the right temporal lobe (Fig. 33U). There is little associated mass effect. The masses show extensive variation in signal intensity, including high and low signal on both T1- and T2-weighted sequences, indicating both T1 and T2 lengthening and shortening.

There are several similar smaller lesions, including a 1.5 cm variable intensity lesion in the left anterior cerebellum (Figs. 33A–C), a small punctate focus of high signal intensity in the right thalamus (Fig. 33T), a small high-intensity focus in the anterior right caudate head (Fig. 33Q), and a 1 cm lesion laterally involving the right frontal lobe cortex (Figs. 33J, K, and P). These lesions also show similar variegated signal intensity.

There has been a previous left temporoparietal craniotomy (Figs. 33G and N), underlying which is a large area of surgical resection of posterior left temporal lobe that is now replaced with cerebrospinal fluid (which is likely to communicate with the atrium of the left lateral ventricle). A left ventricular shunt tube is noted in this region (Fig. 33M), and there is local distortion from metallic artifact at the craniotomy site (Fig. 33M). Anterior to the craniotomy is a small 8 mm chronic epidural collection (Fig. 33I); posterosuperior to the craniotomy site is a 5 mm chronic subdural collection (Fig. 33L).

There is generalized atrophy of the cerebrum and cerebellum with enlargement of the ventricular system and the cerebral and cerebellar sulci. Fluid is present in the left mastoid air cells.

Diagnosis

Multiple cavernous angiomata, cerebral and cerebellar atrophy, and chronic subdural and epidural hematomata.

Discussion

Cavernous angiomata consist of large, dilated, endothelial-lined vascular spaces without intervening brain parenchyma. They are usually angiographically occult, and thrombosis and calcification are frequent. They usually present with seizures (with or without hemorrhage) or slowly evolving focal neurologic deficits, although they may be asymptomatic. They are multiple in up to one-third of cases and may be familial and associated with angiomas of other organs, most often the skin.

Magnetic resonance imaging shows features typical of previous hemorrhage, with subacute methemoglobin components causing T1 shortening and chronic hemosiderin deposition causing T2 shortening and signal loss, which may also be due to associated calcium deposition. The surrounding brain may undergo gliosis. These lesions contain stagnant blood that also has a short T1 and long T2. Of note is the absence of any evidence of enlarged supplying arteries or draining veins, differentiating these lesions from the more common arteriovenous malformations. Gradient echo imaging is useful to detect blood products that cause alterations in local magnetic susceptibility.

References

1. Atlas SW, Mark AS, Fram EK, Grossman RI. Vascular intracranial lesions: applications of gradient echo MR imaging. *Radiology* 1988;169:455–461.
2. Heinz ER. Angiographically occult cerebrovascular malformations and venous angiomas. In: Taveris JM, Ferrucci JT, eds., *Radiology: diagnosis-imaging-intervention,* vol. 3. Philadelphia: Lippincott, 1986;1–6.

Submitted by: Stephen J. Davis, M.D. and Louis M. Teresi, M.D., Huntington Medical Research Institutes, Pasadena, California; William G. Bradley, Jr., M.D., Ph.D., Senior Editor.

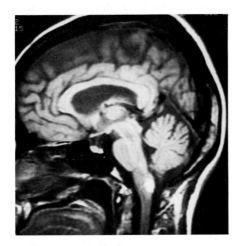

FIG. 34A. SE 800/20.

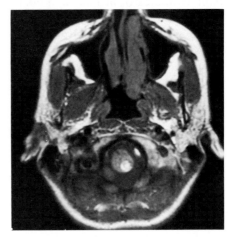

FIG. 34B. SE 800/20.

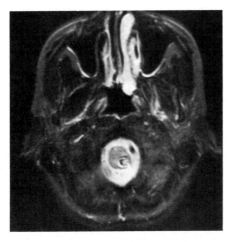

FIG. 34C. SE 2,800/90.

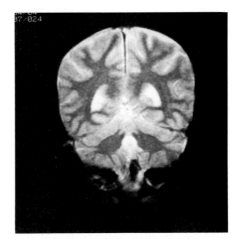

FIG. 34D. GRE 800/15/20°.

Clinical History

Sudden onset of left-sided numbness of the face prompted the MR study of this 41-year-old woman.

Findings

A small, oval area of high signal intensity seen in the dorsal aspect of the medulla on the T1-weighted sagittal (Fig. 34A) and the T1-weighted axial (Fig. 34B) images. The T2-weighted axial (Fig. 34C) and the gradient-recalled coronal (Fig. 34D) images show a preferential signal loss within the lesion. Note the minimal mass effect and the lack of surrounding edema.

Diagnosis

Surgically confirmed cavernous angioma.

Discussion

Four general categories of vascular malformation afflict the brain. High-flow arteriovenous malformations are characterized by large feeding vessels to a network of arteriolar and capillary shunts, leading to large draining veins. These are generally angiographically detectable and easily seen on MR as prominent collections of serpentine structures with signal void. Two histologic types of angiographically occult vascular malformations also appear in the brain. The first, cavernous angioma, is a collection of enlarged capillary spaces with no intervening brain tissue between them. The second is a capillary telangiectasia which is a proliferation of capillaries at the microscopic level, with some interspersed brain tissue. The latter two lesions may present with hemorrhage, but, more often, their clinical presentation is that of headaches or seizures. They may be incidentally discovered. The history of these lesions is one of repetitive, small bleeds. Therefore, the MR image may show evidence of recent as well as old hemorrhage (methemoglobin paramagnetic effect in the center, hemosiderin magnetic susceptibility effect in the periphery). Computed tomography may show calcification. Little, if any, edema is generally seen. The lesion size may increase over time.

In this particular case, the appearance is a rather non-specific one of recent hemorrhage, with the methemoglobin paramagnetic effect predominating on the T1-weighted images, while the magnetic susceptibility effect of intracellular deoxyhemoglobin and/or methemoglobin is shown on the T2-weighted and gradient-recalled images. Therefore, the differential diagnosis would be that of spontaneous bleeding into the medulla due to hypertensive insult (somewhat unusual in a 41-year-old individual), into a tumor such as glioma (unusual in this location), or into a metastatic focus such as melanoma or other highly vascular small metastatic lesion. Given the absence of other lesions, metastatic disease is less likely. The ultimate diagnosis rests on surgical biopsy in cases in which the hemorrhage is recent. If low-signal peripheral hemosiderin effect can be detected indicating old prior bleed in the same location, the diagnosis of an occult arteriovenous vascular malformation would be more certain.

Finally, the symptomatology of facial numbness most likely reflects the effect of the lesion on the descending tract and the nucleus of the 5th nerve, which can be found in this general location. The spinothalamic tract coursing cephalad in this area is responsible for a contralateral altered sensation.

References

1. Gomori J, et al. NMR relaxation times of blood: dependence on field strength, oxidation state, and cell integrity. *J Comput Assist Tomogr* 1987;11:684–690.
2. Lemme-Plaghos L. MR imaging of angiographically occult vascular malformations. *AJNR* 1986;7:217–222.
3. Sze G, et al. Hemorrhagic neoplasms: MR mimics of occult vascular malformations. *AJR* 1987;149:1223–1230.
4. Naseen M, et al. Cervical medullary hematoma: diagnosis by MR. *AJNR* 1986;7:1096–1098.
5. Rigamontid, et al. The MRI appearance of cavernous malformations. *J Neurosurg* 1987;67:518–524.

Submitted by: Roger Bird, M.D., Barrow's Institute, Phoenix, Arizona; Michael Brant-Zawadzki, M.D., Senior Editor.

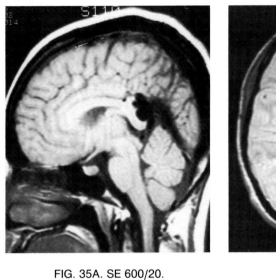

FIG. 35A. SE 600/20.

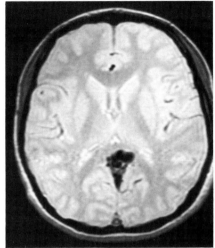

FIG. 35B. SE 2,800/30.

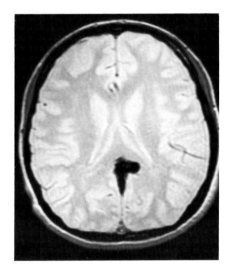

FIG. 35C. SE 2,800/30.

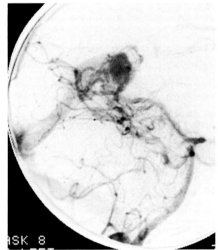

FIG. 35D. Angiogram.

Clinical History

A 33-year-old woman with sudden onset of headache and vomiting.

Findings

The T1-weighted sagittal image (Fig. 35A) shows a bulbous lesion posterior to the splenium of the corpus callosum with low signal intensity characteristics. The first echo images (Figs. 35B and C) of the T2-weighted sequence show a multi-lobulated lesion with very low signal intensity; the lower level shows a rather prominent serpentine structure entering the lower portion of the lesion (Fig. 35C). Note the absence of any high signal intensity on the T1-weighted images surrounding the lesion, or any edema on the T2-weighted axial sequences.

The angiogram (Fig. 35D) verifies the arteriovenous malformation of the posterior corpus callosum with a venous varix simulating a vein of Galen aneurysm.

The GRASS sequence shows the flow phase phenomenon through the brain from the lesion, although the very rapid nature of the flow in the lesion maintains high-velocity signal loss in the lesion despite the gradient-echo technique of this particular study (Fig. 35E).

Diagnosis

Arteriovenous malformation.

Discussion

Two types of "vein of Galen" aneurysm arteriovenous malformations exist. The first is congenital and presents in infancy, usually with congestive failure. This is due to a malformation of the vein of Galen wall. Multiple feeding vessels, generally parenchymal, contribute to this type of lesion, which produces a giant varix of the vein of Galen and very rapid shunting into the straight sinus, accounting for the progressive congestive failure.

The second type of vein of Galen malformation can be seen in adulthood, as in this case, and represents an acquired lesion. It generally occurs when the vein of Galen or one of its tributaries becomes enlarged in varicose fashion due to a nearby malformation that drains into this structure.

References

1. Mills, et al. Nuclear magnetic resonance: principles of blood flow imaging. *AJNR* 1983;4:1161–1167.
2. Bradley W, et al. The appearance of rapidly flowing blood on magnetic resonance images. *AJR* 1984;143:1167–1174.
3. Bradley W, et al. The flow phenomena in MR imaging. *AJR* 1988;150:983–994.
4. Worthington B, et al. NMR imaging in the recognition of giant intracranial aneurysms. *AJNR* 1983;4:835–836.

Submitted by: Michael Brant-Zawadzki, M.D., Senior Editor.

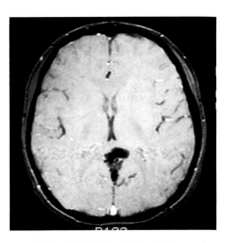

FIG. 35E. GRE 250/15/50°.

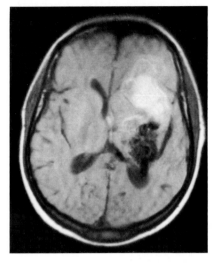 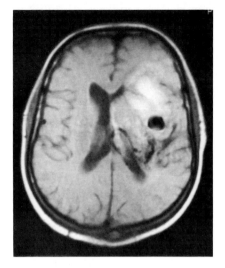

FIG. 36A. SE 1,000/26.   FIG. 36B. SE 1,000/26.

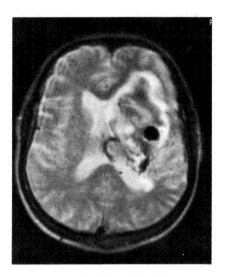

FIG. 36C. SE 2,500/100.

Clinical History

Sudden hemiplegia and aphasia in a 60-year-old man.

Findings

The T1-weighted images (Figs. 36A and B) reveal a striking lesion in the left deep temporal lobe and basal ganglia. A network of serpentine structures is seen immediately anterior to the atrium of the left ventricular system (Fig. 36A), with high signal collection anterior. The higher slice (Fig. 36B) reveals a globular region of signal void in the posterior edge of the high-signal abnormality. Midline shift is seen, as is left ventricular compression. The T2-weighted image (Fig. 36C) verifies the low signal of the spherical lesion shown in Fig. 36B. The high-signal collection anterior to this lesion has become isointense to low in signal intensity, with a border of high signal intensity shown as well.

The angiogram in Fig. 36D verifies the presence of a prominent arteriovenous malformation with an aneurysmal varix at the anterior border, presumably the source of hemorrhage shown in the MR images.

Diagnosis

Arteriovenous malformation with acute hemorrhage and aneurysmal varix.

Discussion

Magnetic resonance offers a potent combination of sensitivity to flow effects, as well as hemorrhagic by-products, which enables accurate evaluation of intracranial intravenous malformations. The time-of-flight phenomena, as well as spine phase changes, which produce the characteristic appearance of blood vessels, enable the network of the arteriovenous malformation to be well visualized. Complicating aneurysms, which can occur in approximately 5–10% of all patients with arteriovenous malformations, can be identified when these are sufficiently large. The ability to detect hemorrhage, and even date its onset, is of importance in deciding on patient management. Arteriovenous malformations that have not hemorrhaged are generally treated more conservatively than ones that can be documented to have blood. Clinical signs and/or symptoms are sometimes inconclusive in the latter category of patients.

Note the relatively low signal of the fresh clot in this case studied at 0.5 T. Clot retraction and fibrin deposition are non–field-dependent mechanisms that contribute to T2 relaxation shortening, which is accentuated by magnetic susceptibility effects, particularly at high fields.

References

1. Smith HJ, Strother M, Kikuchi Y. MR imaging in the management of supratentorial intracranial arteriovenous malformations. *Am J Radiol* 1988;9:225–235.
2. Spetzler RF, Martin NA. A proposed grading system for arteriovenous malformations. *J Neurosurg* 1986;65:476–483.

Submitted by: Michael Brant-Zawadzki, M.D., Senior Editor.

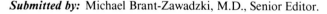

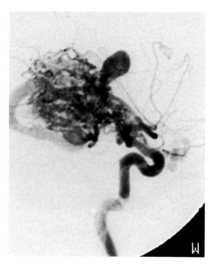

FIG. 36D. Angiogram.

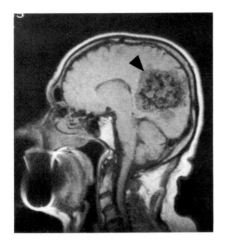

FIG. 37A. SE 500/35.

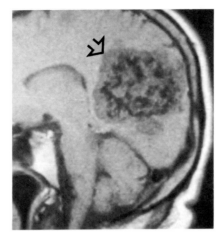

FIG. 37B. SE 500/35.

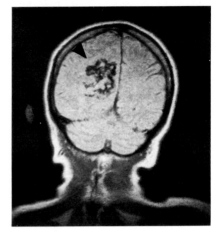

FIG. 37C. SE 1,500/35.

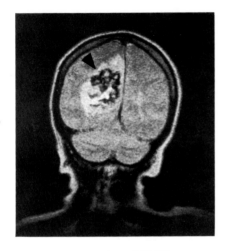

FIG. 37D. SE 1,500/70.

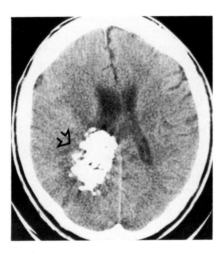

FIG. 37E. CT.

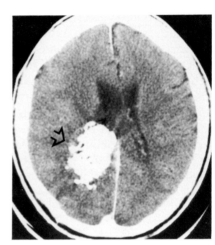

FIG. 37F. CT with contrast.

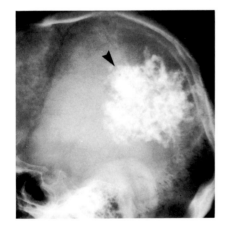

FIG. 37G. Plain film.

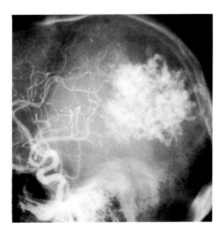

FIG. 37H. Angiogram.

Clinical History

A 16-year-old boy with seizures.

Findings

Coronal proton-density and T2-weighted (SE 1,500/35 and 70) and sagittal T1-weighted (SE 500/35) images are provided for review. Non-enhanced and enhanced CT, plain film, and angiograms are also provided. The sagittal SE 500/35 image shows an intermediate-signal mass in the right posterior-parietal lobe (Fig. 37A, *arrow*). A magnified view of the mass (Fig. 37B, *open arrow*) shows the numerous irregular/rounded signal-void elements within the intermediate signal mass. The SE 1,500/35 coronal image shows only the signal-void internal architecture, which, in this plane, has a serpiginous appearance (Fig. 37C, *arrowhead*). The SE 1,500/70 coronal image shows a high-intensity mass with serpiginous signal-void internal architecture (Fig. 37D, *arrowhead*). Non-contrast CT shows dense calcification in the mass (Fig. 37E, *open arrow*) and contrast-enhanced CT reveals no contrast enhancement (Fig. 37F, *open arrow*). Lateral plain film shows the dense "cloud" of calcifications to best advantage (Fig. 37G, *arrowhead*), and internal carotid angiogram shows no neovascularity (Fig. 37H).

Diagnosis

Thrombosed cavernous hemangioma.

Discussion

Cavernous angiomas are composed of large sinusoidal vascular spaces that are closely clustered together. Unlike arteriovenous malformations (AVMs), the vessels are not separated by normal neural tissue. Angiomas represent the rarest form of vascular malformation but are clinically important because they are often symptomatic, causing seizures. They are commonly within the cerebral hemispheres, particularly in the subcortical region. Calcification is present in 30% of cases secondary to partial or complete thrombosis. Angiography is frequently normal, although prolonged injection angiography may demonstrate feeding arteries, a capillary blush, and abnormal draining veins. Computed tomography findings consist of a hyperdense and often partially calcified lesion that shows fairly homogeneous enhancement of minimal degree or no enhancement.

On MR images, cavernous angiomas appear as well-defined, rounded lesions, hyperintense on T2-weighted images, with lesion heterogeneity related to calcification and a relatively complex matrix. Those with dense calcification may appear nearly signal void. They may contain foci of hemorrhage with resultant intensity variations dependent on the age of the hemorrhage. Mild mass effect may be noted with acute or subacute hemorrhage. More typically, the lack of mass effect or changes over serial examinations should suggest the diagnosis. Unlike AVMs, cavernous angiomas do not show enlarged feeding or draining vessels.

Reference

1. Lee BC, Herzberg L, Zimmerman RD, et al. MR imaging of cerebral vascular malformations. *AJNR* 1985;6:863–870.

Submitted by: Louis M. Teresi, M.D. and Stephen J. Davis, M.D., Huntington Medical Research Institutes, Pasadena, California; William G. Bradley, Jr., M.D., Ph.D., Senior Editor.

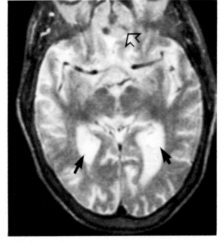

FIG. 38A. SE 3,000/40.

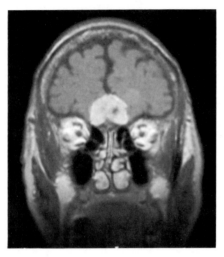

FIG. 38B. SE 3,000/80.

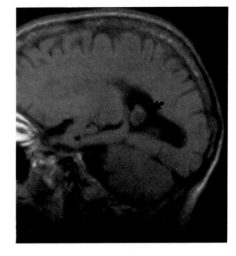

FIG. 38C. SE 750/30.

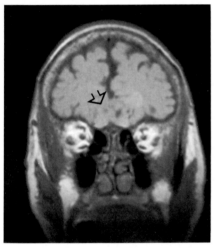

FIG. 38D. SE 750/30.

FIG. 38E. SE 750/30 with Gd-DTPA.

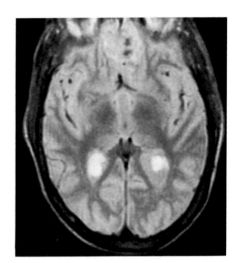

FIG. 38F. SE 3,000/40.

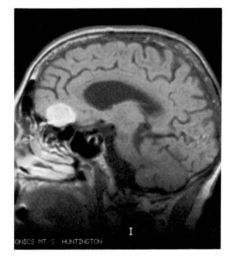

FIG. 38G. SE 750/30 with Gd-DTPA.

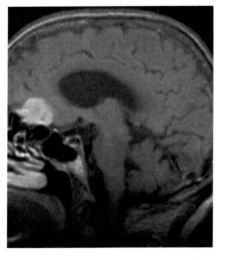

FIG. 38H. SE 750/30 with Gd-DTPA.

Clinical History

This 75-year-old woman was noted to have downbeat nystagmus during a routine eye check-up.

Findings

A 4 cm midline extra-axial mass arises from the region of the cribiform plate surrounding the inferior falx bilaterally. This mass is relatively isointense with respect to gray matter on both T1- and T2-weighted sequences and has multiple punctate foci of low signal within it, representing foci of calcification (Figs. 38A, B, and D, *open arrows*). Following gadolinium, there is diffuse, homogeneous contrast enhancement (Figs. 38E, G, and H). The features are typical of a meningioma.

There are bilateral rounded and lobulated masses of the choroid plexus in the atria of both lateral ventricles, measuring 2 cm on the right and 1.5 cm on the left. These masses are of high signal intensity on T2-weighted sequences (Figs. 38A and B, *arrows*) and do not show contrast enhancement following gadolinium (Fig. 38C, *arrow*).

There is a moderate degree of atrophy involving both cerebral hemispheres and the pons. Scattered foci of high signal intensity in the deep white matter represent mild ischemic changes. There is a small retention cyst in the left maxillary sinus.

Diagnosis

Xanthogranulomata of the choroid plexus and subfrontal meningioma.

Discussion

The features of the meningioma are typical and are discussed elsewhere. The bilateral choroid plexus lesions represent xanthogranulomata of the choroid plexus and are an incidental finding of no clinical significance. The features in this case are typical, with T1 shortening relative to cerebrospinal fluid and no contrast enhancement. There may be a peripheral rim of low signal, corresponding to a rim of calcification seen on CT scans. Xanthogranulomata are incidental findings that should be differentiated from rare intraventricular meningiomas, which typically enhance with gadolinium and may cause some localized obstruction of the temporal horn and choroid plexus papillomas. The choroid plexus papillomas also typically enhance and often show multiple vascular channels of flow void within the mass on MR. Angiomatous abnormalities associated with the Sturge-Weber syndrome may also affect the choroid plexus, but these contrast enhance as well. All of these lesions are usually unilateral, in contrast to the bilateral changes of xanthogranulomata.

Xanthogranulomata of the choroid plexus are characterized pathologically as variable-size masses with lipid deposits, neuroepithelial microcysts, and peripheral psammoma body calcifications. In a group of 167 patients, Hinshaw et al. (1) found that approximately 40% of patients had bright choroid plexus glomera. Of those patients who had CT scans, the typical CT appearance of these bright glomera consisted of non-enhancing central regions of low (but not negative) attenuation, with peripheral calcifications in the majority. The remainder showed noncalcified glomera.

Reference

1. Hinshaw DB, Fahmy JL, Peckham N, et al. Abnormal choroid plexus on MR: CT and pathological correlation. *AJNR* 1988;9:483–496.

Submitted by: Stephen J. Davis, M.D., Louis M. Teresi, M.D., and Mark Ziemba, M.D., Huntington Medical Research Institutes, Pasadena, California; William G. Bradley, Jr., M.D., Ph.D., Senior Editor.

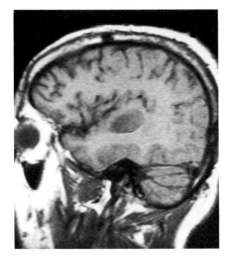

FIG. 40A. November 7, 1987, SE 600/20.

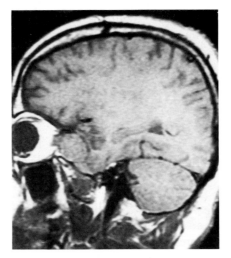

FIG. 40B. November 7, 1987, SE 600/20.

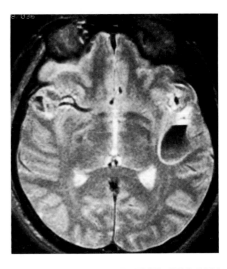

FIG. 40C. November 7, 1987, SE 2,800/ 70.

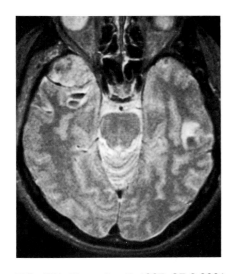

FIG. 40D. November 7, 1987, SE 2,800/ 70.

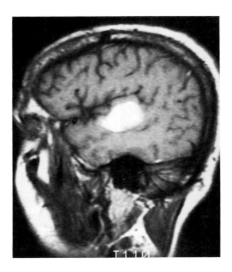

FIG. 40E. December 4, 1987, SE 600/20.

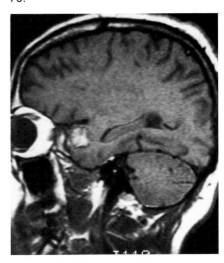

FIG. 40F. December 4, 1987, SE 600/20.

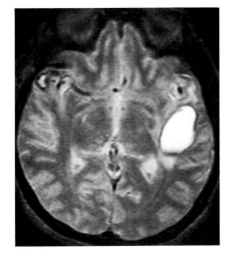

FIG. 40G. December 4, 1987, SE 2,800/ 70.

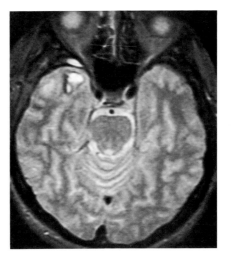

FIG. 40H. December 4, 1987, SE 2,800/ 70.

Clinical History

A 44-year-old man fell during a drinking bout. Linear temporal fracture prompted CT and MR scanning.

Findings

The initial T1-weighted sagittal images demonstrate the left sylvian region hematoma as a low signal intensity focal collection (Fig. 40A), whereas the epidural hematoma (suffered at the same time) is seen as isointense (Fig. 40B). Immediately posterior to the epidural, low-intensity contusions are apparent within the right temporal lobe as well. The signal intensity of the left sylvian hematoma is quite low on the T2-weighted image, with a fluid-fluid level seen. The supernatant is quite bright. The dependent red blood cell layer is quite dark due to signal reflecting the intracellular methemoglobin/deoxyhemoglobin and resulting magnetic susceptibility effects. The smaller hemorrhagic contusions of the right temporal lobe also show low signal intensity. Note that the epidural collection anterior to the right temporal lobe (Fig. 40D) remains relatively isointense. Whether this reflects the relatively better perfused dural/epidural space and resultant maintenance of oxyhemoglobin, or some other factor, such as continued bleeding into the epidural space, is not known.

The scan obtained three weeks later shows the left sylvian hematoma as high in signal intensity on the T1-weighted image, reflecting the conversion to methemoglobin in solution (the red blood cells having lysed) (Figs. 40E and F). The epidural hematoma has been surgically removed in the interval. The T2-weighted image persists in showing the elevated signal intensity of the left sylvian hematoma as well as the remnant right temporal contusions (Figs. 40G and H).

Finally, given the patient's persistent difficulty in speech, the left sylvian hematoma was removed. Follow-up scan obtained four weeks later shows the residual hemosiderin effect in the sylvian region as a lowered signal intensity (Fig. 40I).

Diagnosis

Right temporal epidural and temporal intracranial hematomas with evolution and surgery.

Discussion

This case summarizes the typical evolution of acute hemorrhage in the brain substance over time and makes the point that blood collections in different spaces or undergoing different physiologic events may show a different type of signal and evolution. It should be noted that the magnetic properties of blood by-products make MR a more sensitive modality for evaluating posttraumatic syndromes compared with CT scanning.

References

1. Bradley W, et al. Effective methemoglobin formation on the MR appearance of hemorrhage. *Radiology* 1985;156:99–103.
2. Sipponen N, et al. Nuclear magnetic resonance imaging of intracerebral hemorrhage in the acute and resolving phases. *J Comput Assist Tomogr* 1983;7:954–959.
3. Gomori J, et al. Mechanisms responsible for the MR appearance and evolution of intracranial hemorrhage. *Radiographics* 1988;8:427–453.
4. Hesselink J, et al. MR imaging of brain contusions: a comparative study with CT. *AJNR* 1988;9:269–278.

Submitted by: Michael Brant-Zawadzki, M.D., Senior Editor.

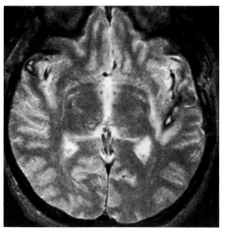

FIG. 40I. January 19, 1988, SE 3,000/70.

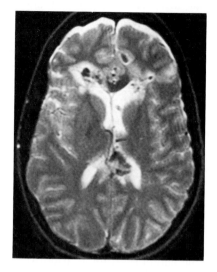

FIG. 42A. SE 2,800/90.

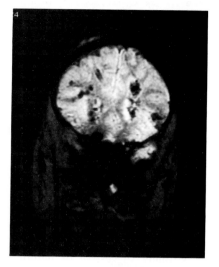

FIG. 42B. GRE 800/35/15°.

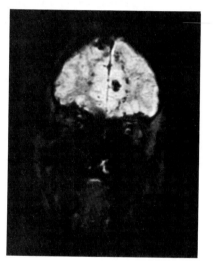

FIG. 42C. GRE 800/35/15°.

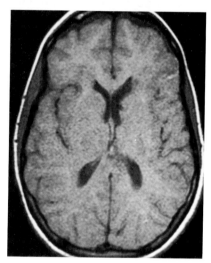

FIG. 42D. SE 800/20.

Clinical History

An 18-year-old with mental dysfunction following a car accident (roll-over) four days prior to MRI.

Findings

Multiple areas of signal loss are scattered throughout the periventricular region. Most notable is the abnormality of the rostrum of the corpus callosum as well as the splenium (Fig. 42A), seen on the T2-weighted axial image. The coronal gradient-echo images show to much better advantage the multiple foci of abnormalities scattered throughout the gray-white matter junctional region (Figs. 42B and C). Peripheral high signal is seen associated with the low-signal foci. Note the absence of significant signal alteration on the corresponding T1-weighted image (Fig. 42D).

Diagnosis

Multiple hemorrhagic contusions, "shear" diffuse brain injury.

Discussion

High-field MRI, particularly gradient-echo imaging, accentuates the magnetic susceptibility effect of recent hemorrhage due to any etiology. The distribution in this patient is quite typical for the presence of rotational forces that produce shear stresses on the brain parenchyma. Since the brain lacks structural rigidity, when the skull is rapidly rotated, the brain lags behind, causing axial stretching, separation, and disruption along borders of disparate density (such as gray and white matter). Such shear injuries commonly can occur in the corpus callosum, a component that may result from contusion against the more rigid flax.

Magnetic resonance is more sensitive than CT for detecting brain contusions. T2-weighted spin-echo images are best for demonstrating such abnormalities. The hemorrhagic component can be accentuated by the gradient-echo sequence, particularly important prior to the methemoglobin stage, which would be seen as high in signal on the T1-weighted sequence.

References

1. Hesselink J, et al. MR imaging of brain contusions, a comparative study with CT. *AJNR* 1988;9:269–278.
2. Han J, et al. Head trauma evaluated by magnetic resonance and computed tomography—a comparison. *Radiology* 1984;150:71–77.
3. Zimmerman R, et al. Head injury: early results of comparing CT and high field MR. *AJNR* 1986;7:757–764.
4. Adams J, et al. Diffuse brain damage of immediate impact type. *Brain* 1977;100:489–502.
5. Holbourn A. Mechanisms of head injuries. *Lancet* 1943;2:438–441.

Submitted by: Roger Bird, M.D., Barrow's Institute, Phoenix, Arizona; Michael Brant-Zawadzki, M.D., Senior Editor.

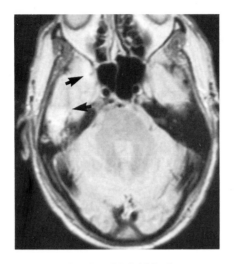 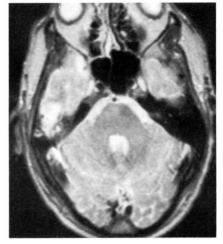

FIG. 43A. SE 3,000/40.   FIG. 43B. SE 3,000/80.

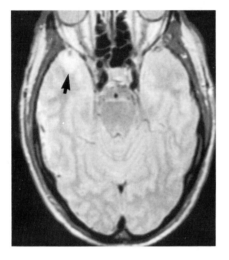 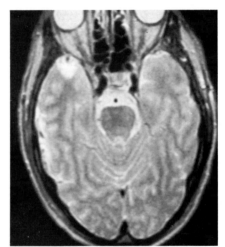

FIG. 43C. SE 3,000/40.   FIG. 43D. SE 3,000/80.

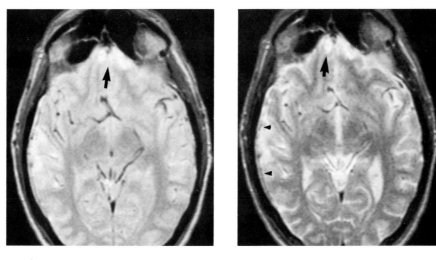

FIG. 43E. SE 3,000/40.   FIG. 43F. SE 3,000/80.

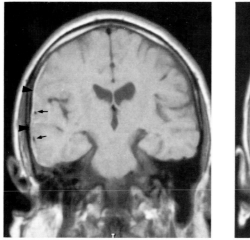
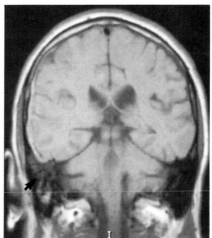

FIG. 43G. SE 500/30.   FIG. 43H. SE 500/30.

Clinical History

A 50-year-old man who, 4 days prior, had tripped and fallen in a parking lot, hitting his head on the concrete.

Findings

T2-weighted axial images show multiple regions of increased signal intensity within the right temporal lobe, particularly within the temporal tip, adjacent to the petrous ridge and superficially (Figs. 43A–D, *arrows*). There are similar lesions involving the superficial aspects of both anterior frontal lobes, particularly immediately above the floor of the anterior cranial fossa (Figs. 43E and F, *arrows*).

There is a thin subdural fluid collection (Figs. 43F and G, *arrowheads*) overlying the right hemisphere, with increased signal intensity on both T1- and T2-weighted sequences and inward displacement of the underlying cortical veins (Fig. 43G, *arrows*). The right mastoid air cells are opacified (Fig. 43H, *arrow*).

Diagnosis

Cerebral contusions involving the right temporal and both frontal lobes, thin right subacute subdural hematoma, and probable right petrous fracture.

Discussion

The distribution of cerebral contusions is determined to a large extent by the shape of the skull, and they are most commonly found adjacent to the roughened bone lining the floor of the anterior cranial fossa, sphenoid wings, and petrous ridges. Tissue injury results in increased vascular permeability and progressive increase in tissue water content, and, in more serious injuries, vascular disruption with hemorrhage occurs, forming hemorrhagic contusions. With nonhemorrhagic contusions, focal areas of prolongation of both T1 and T2 accompanied by possible mass effect are shown, increasing over the first few days and then slowly resolving. The result of these lesions is areas of encephalomalacia with varying degrees of sulcal prominence and focal ventricular dilatation. The first observable MR evidence of hemorrhage can be seen 12–24 hours after the injury and is manifested as areas of T2 shortening, representing intracellular deoxyhemoglobin. In chronic hemorrhagic lesions, changes demonstrating either T1 shortening due to methemoglobin formation or T2 shortening due to hemosiderin formation have been shown. Evidence of hemosiderin formation in a rim around the hematoma has been seen as early as three days following injury.

These findings are in contrast to the CT findings, in which hemorrhage can be seen as an area of increased density within one hour of injury and the decreased attenuation due to encephalomalacia is seen several weeks later. Magnetic resonance is more sensitive in detecting posterior fossa and temporal lobe lesions and in demonstrating the subacute and chronic effects of the hemorrhage. Computed tomography remains a sensitive modality for detecting early parenchymal and subarachnoid hemorrhage.

Subdural hematomas show three distinct MR appearances as they age. Acute subdural hematomas are characterized by low intensity on T2-weighted images, particularly with high-field units. This is due to the selective T2 shortening caused by deoxyhemoglobin within intact red blood cells and is seen within the first week following injury. Subacute subdural collections are characterized by high signal on T1-weighted images and are subdivided into early subacute (red blood cells intact), where the signal intensity is low on T2-weighted images, and late subacute (red blood cells lysed), where the signal intensity is high on T2-weighted images. These changes are similar to those seen in parenchymal hematomas and are due to the paramagnetic effects of methemoglobin. However, the changes in chronic subdural hematomas differ from intraparenchymal bleeds. Chronic subdurals appear slightly hypointense to isointense on short TR/TE images with loss of the T1 shortening from a decrease in the concentration of free methemoglobin. Unlike parenchymal hematomas, a rim of hemosiderin manifesting as hypointensity on long TR/TE sequences is uncommon in chronic subdural hematomas, although it can be seen in thickened membranes in patients who have rehemorrhaged. Inward displacement of the cortical veins is a useful sign to differentiate chronic subdural collections from enlarged cerebrospinal fluid spaces.

References

1. Fobbenes, Grossman RI, Atlas SW, et al. MR characteristics of subdural hematomas and hygromas at 1.5 T. *AJR* 1989;153:589–595.
2. Hesselink JR, Dowd CF, Healy ME. MR imaging of brain contusions: a comparative study with CT. *AJNR* 1988;9:269–278.

Submitted by: Stephen J. Davis, M.D., Louis M. Teresi, M.D., and Mark Ziemba, M.D., Huntington Medical Research Institutes, Pasadena, California; William G. Bradley, Jr., M.D., Ph.D., Senior Editor.

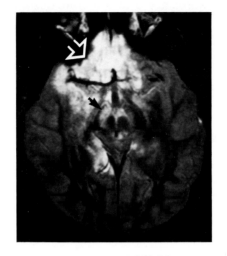

FIG. 44A. SE 2,800/30.

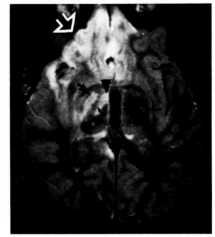

FIG. 44B. SE 2,800/30.

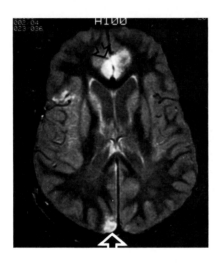

FIG. 44C. SE 2,800/30.

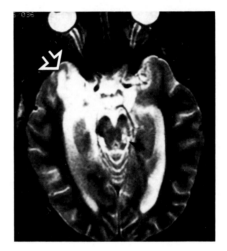

FIG. 44D. SE 2,800/90.

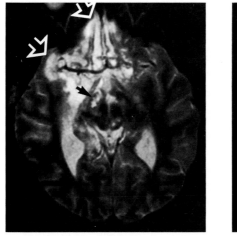

FIG. 44E. SE 2,800/90.

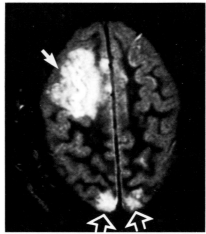

FIG. 44F. SE 2,800/30.

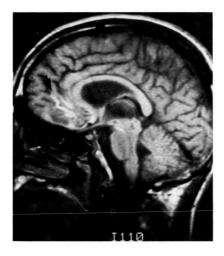

FIG. 44G. SE 800/20.

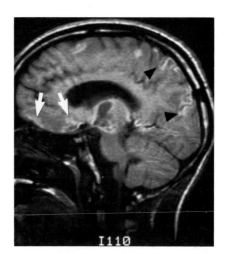

FIG. 44H. SE 800/20.

Clinical History

A 16-year-old man who was involved in a high-velocity motor vehicle accident eight weeks previously.

111

Findings

Axial T2-weighted and sagittal T1-weighted images are provided for review. The axial T2-weighted images (Figs. 44A–F) show large regions of increased signal intensity in the right and left frontal lobes (Figs. 44A, B, and E, *open arrows*), right temporal lobe (Fig. 44D, *open arrow*), high right frontoparietal lobe (Fig. 44F, *arrow*), and in the posterior aspects of both occipital lobes (Fig. 44F, *open arrows*). These regions of increased signal intensity involve both the gray and white matter.

Increased signal is also seen in the right cerebral peduncle (Fig. 44E, *arrow*), left lateral midbrain tegmentum (Fig. 44D, *arrow*), right thalamus (Fig. 44B, *arrowhead*), and lenticular nucleus (Fig. 44B, *large arrow*), sparing the internal capsule (Fig. 44B, *small arrow*).

The sagittal T1-weighted image shows high signal within the callosomarginal sulcus (Fig. 44G, *arrow*), floor of the anterior cranial fossa (Fig. 44H, *arrows*), and superficial cortical sulci of the posterior parietal and occipital lobes (Fig. 44H, *arrowheads*). A prominent cerebrospinal fluid (CSF) flow void is seen in the 3rd ventricle (Fig. 44B, *crossed arrow*), aqueduct, and 4th ventricle on the SE 2,800/30 image.

Diagnosis

Coup-contrecoup posttraumatic edema, subarachnoid hemorrhage, communicating hydrocephalus, and brainstem shear injury.

Discussion

Several mechanisms can be responsible for brain injury; however, the best known is the coup-contrecoup injury. In this mechanism of injury, the skull comes to an abrupt stop, but the brain continues to move. The brain then comes to an abrupt stop against the inner table of the calvarium. That part of the brain located opposite the impact site is cavitated from being pulled suddenly from its dura. Injury to the brain at the primary impact site is referred to as the coup injury; that on the opposite side is referred to as the contrecoup. Sites of predilection of brain injury are those regions where the moving brain may be sheared or impacted on the inner table: inferior surface of the frontal lobe, temporal pole, occipital pole, and rolandic convexity.

Traumatized brain parenchyma becomes edematous over the hours or days following injury. Vasogenic edema is moderately hypointense on T1-weighted images and very hyperintense on T2-weighted images. Edema occurs at the site of injury and spreads into the surrounding white matter in a pseudopod-like fashion, tending to spare the non-injured areas and overlying cortex. Edema is easily shown and separated from hemorrhagic cortex in the acute head injury patients on T2-weighted images. After the edema resolves, hyperintensity frequently remains secondary to gliosis. The result years later may be encephalomalacia, with varying degrees of sulcal prominence and ventricular dilatation.

Shearing injuries result in local hemorrhage or edema in both white and gray matter. The most common locations for shearing injuries are the subcortical gray-white matter interfaces, the upper pons and midbrain, the internal capsule, and the corpus callosum.

Subarachnoid hemorrhage (SAH), frequently found in patients with head injury, has a variable appearance on MR images depending on the oxidative state of hemoglobin. As in this case, the presence of methemoglobin in subacute hemorrhage causes high signal on both T1- and T2-weighted images.

Subarachnoid hemorrhage may lead to communicating hydrocephalus as a result of obstruction of the CSF resorption pathways, usually the arachnoid villi. The arachnoid villi are normally responsible for the uptake of CSF, which is drained into the venous system via the superior sagittal sinus. Less commonly, noncommunicating hydrocephalus may develop acutely secondary to hemorrhage within the ventricular system or around the aqueduct, obstructing ventricular pathways. The latter develops more rapidly than that due to extraventricular obstruction.

The diagnosis of communicating hydrocephalus can be made if there is ventricular dilatation without sulcal enlargement. Magnetic resonance has proved most useful in the diagnosis of the hyperdynamic CSF flow state associated with communicating hydrocephalus. The intensity of the CSF in the aqueduct is generally less than in the lateral ventricles due to its back and forth motion through the aqueduct during the cardiac cycle. The pulsatile flow of CSF in the aqueduct reflects many factors, among them the ventricular surface area and the sclerosis or compression of cortical veins (which are unable to vent venous blood during diastole). Although this aqueductal flow void can be seen in normal patients, it is much more prominent in patients with chronic communicating hydrocephalus and normal pressure hydrocephalus, and extends into the adjacent 4th and 3rd ventricles. On mildly T2-weighted images, the greatest signal loss is seen in patients with chronic communicating hydrocephalus, and the least is seen in patients with obstructive hydrocephalus and atrophy.

References

1. Kelly AB, Zimmerman RD, Snow RB, et al. Head trauma: comparison of MR and CT-experience in 100 patients. *AJNR* 1988;9:699–708.
2. Hesselink JR, Dowd CF, Healy ME, et al. MR imaging of brain contusions: a comparative study with CT. *AJNR* 1988;9:269–278.
3. Gentry LR, Godersky JC, Thompson BH. Traumatic brainstem injury: MR imaging. *Radiology* 1989;171:177–187.
4. Bradley WG, Kortman KE, Burgoyne R. Flowing cerebrospinal fluid in normal and hydrocephalic states: appearance on MR images. *Radiology* 1986;159:611–616.

Submitted by: Louis M. Teresi, M.D., Stephen J. Davis, M.D., and Mark Ziemba, M.D., Huntington Medical Research Institutes, Pasadena, California; William G. Bradley, Jr., M.D., Ph.D., Senior Editor.

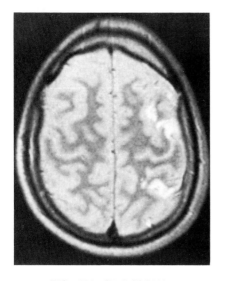

FIG. 45A. SE 3,000/40.

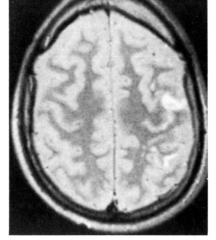

FIG. 45B. SE 3,000/40.

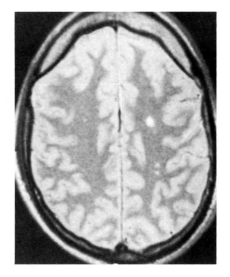

FIG. 45C. SE 3,000/40.

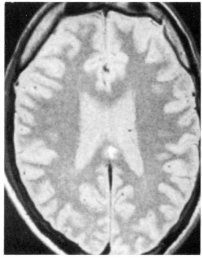

FIG. 45D. SE 3,000/40.

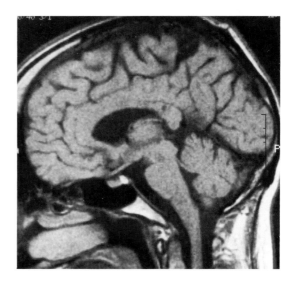

FIG. 45E. SE 500/40.

Clinical History

Numbness of the right side of the face following head injury in a motor vehicle accident one month prior to the scan.

Findings

Axial 5 mm proton density-weighted (SE 3,000/40) and sagittal 5 mm T1-W (SE 500/40) images are presented. There are multiple predominantly subcortical (Figs. 45A and B) lesions in the left posterior frontal and parietal lobes situated at the corticomedullary junction. There is also a vertically oriented 7 mm diameter lesion extending through the white matter of the corona radiata of the posterior frontal lobe on the left, extending toward the lateral ventricle (Fig. 45C). A further irregular 1 cm lesion is present involving the splenium of the corpus callosum (Figs. 45D and E). No brainstem lesion is evident, and there is no evidence of an extra-axial collection or MR evidence of hemorrhage. Thickening of the diploic space of the frontal bone is noted bilaterally.

Diagnosis

Shearing injury involving the left cerebral hemisphere and corpus callosum.

Discussion

Shearing injury or "diffuse axonal injury" is mediated through shear-strain forces generated by rotational acceleration of the head. Diffuse axonal injury from rotation typically occurs in the cerebral white matter, the corpus callosum, and the dorsolateral quadrants of the rostral brainstem. These lesions are usually nonhemorrhagic, tend to be multiple, typically vary from 5 to 15 mm in size, and are characteristically distributed at the gray-white matter interface, the white matter of the corona radiata, and the splenium of the corpus callosum. The majority are located at the gray-white interface in the frontal and temporal lobes and the subjacent corona radiata. Corpus callosal lesions are usually slightly off midline or bilateral and may be associated with intraventricular hemorrhage. The internal capsule is not commonly involved; if so, it is usually at the junction with the cerebral peduncle. Approximately 20% of these lesions have evidence of hemorrhage. Diffuse axonal injury is more often present with initial impairment of consciousness, although this is not necessarily so.

The diffuse thickening of the diploic space in the frontal bone (Figs. 45C and E) should not be mistaken for a subacute subdural hematoma. This may be particularly prominent in patients with hyperostosis frontalis interna.

Reference

1. Gentry LR, Godersky JC, Thompson B. MR imaging of head trauma: review of the distribution and radiopathological features of traumatic lesion. *AJNR* 1988;9:101–110.

Submitted by: Stephen J. Davis, M.D. and Louis M. Teresi, M.D., Huntington Medical Research Institutes, Pasadena, California; William G. Bradley, Jr., M.D., Ph.D., Senior Editor.

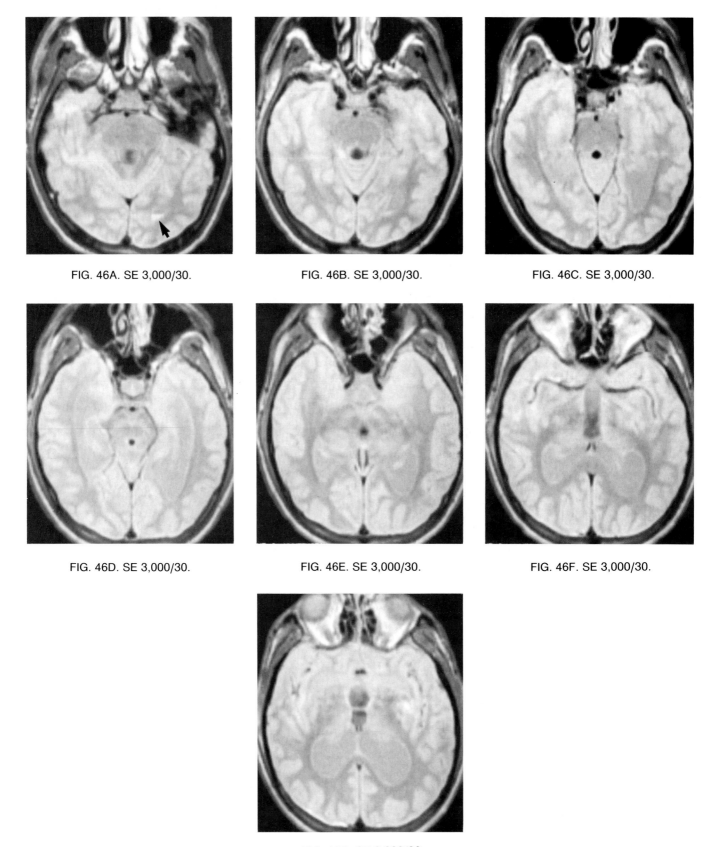

FIG. 46A. SE 3,000/30.

FIG. 46B. SE 3,000/30.

FIG. 46C. SE 3,000/30.

FIG. 46D. SE 3,000/30.

FIG. 46E. SE 3,000/30.

FIG. 46F. SE 3,000/30.

FIG. 46G. SE 3,000/30.

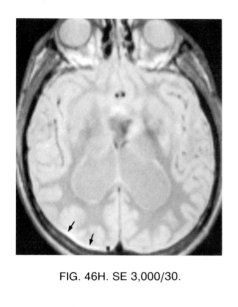

FIG. 46H. SE 3,000/30.

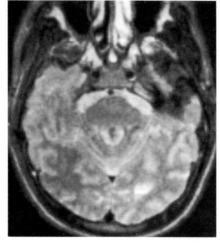

FIG. 46I. SE 3,000/80.

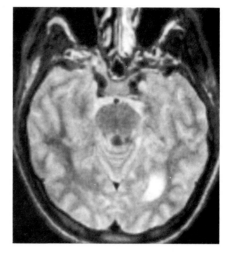

FIG. 46J. SE 3,000/80.

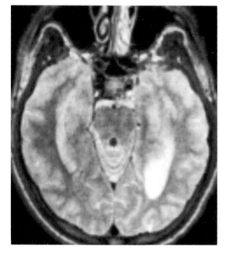

FIG. 46K. SE 3,000/80.

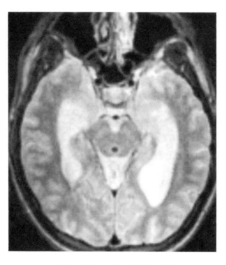

FIG. 46L. SE 3,000/80.

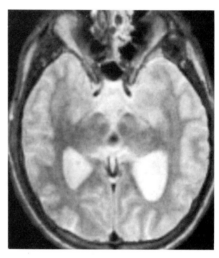

FIG. 46M. SE 3,000/80.

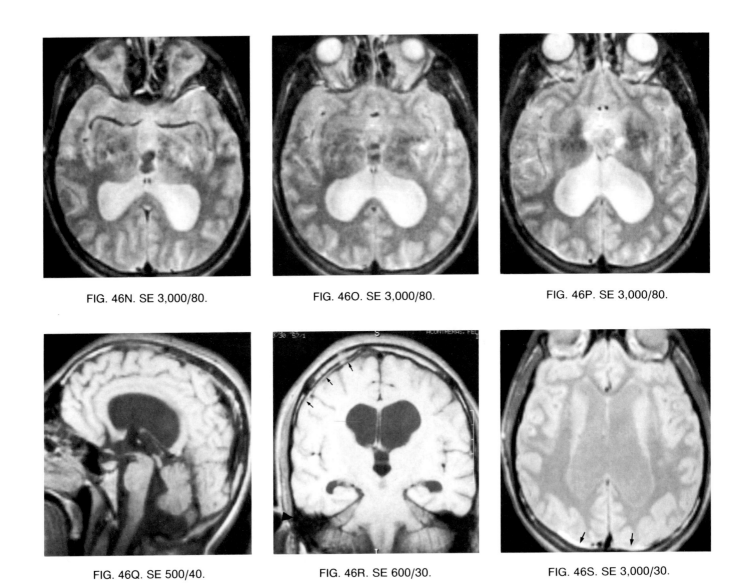

FIG. 46N. SE 3,000/80.

FIG. 46O. SE 3,000/80.

FIG. 46P. SE 3,000/80.

FIG. 46Q. SE 500/40.

FIG. 46R. SE 600/30.

FIG. 46S. SE 3,000/30.

Clinical History

A 22-year-old man who fell from a cliff. He was scanned two days later while still unconscious.

Findings

There is marked enlargement of the ventricles associated with upward bowing of the corpus callosum (Fig. 46Q), with no evidence of dilatation of the cortical sulci. There is a thin rim of high signal intensity surrounding the lateral ventricles on the T2-weighted images. On the axial T2-weighted images, there is prominent cerebrospinal fluid (CSF) signal loss involving the cerebral aqueduct, extending through the 3rd ventricle and then via the foramen of Monro into the anterior horns of the lateral ventricles (Figs. 46A–O). This CSF flow void extends distally into the lower 4th ventricle.

A small fluid-fluid level is present in the dependent portion of the left occipital horn of the lateral ventricle, with the dependent portion being of increased signal intensity (Fig. 46A, *arrow*). There is a thin extra-axial collection overlying both posterior parietal lobes, more marked on the right side, which is of high intensity on both the sagittal T1-weighted and the T2-weighted sequences (Figs. 46H, R, and S, *arrows*).

Punctate areas of high signal intensity involve the inferior left putamen and the paraventricular white matter of the right centrum semiovale. Extensive artifact arising from the turbulent CSF flow within the 3rd ventricle is distributed transversely across the temporal lobe. There is fluid within right mastoid air cells (Fig. 46R, *arrowhead*).

Diagnosis

Posttraumatic communicating hydrocephalus, small bilateral subacute subdural hematomas, and intraventricular hemorrhage.

Discussion

The features are typical of communicating hydrocephalus, in which the obstruction to CSF flow occurs distal to the outlet foramina of the 4th ventricle due to pathologic processes involving the subarachnoid spaces, arachnoid villi, or venous sinuses. It commonly occurs secondary to subarachnoid hemorrhage (SAH) or infectious meningitis. If it develops acutely, it is usually accompanied by headaches, vomiting, papilledema, and obtundation. If the mode of onset is less precipitous, then these symptoms may be absent. Communicating hydrocephalus may develop following trauma as a result of blood in the subarachnoid space. Although SAH is not specifically identified, this is likely to be the cause in this case because the fluid-fluid level seen in the left occipital horn appears to be due to blood products, particularly in view of the bilateral small subdural hematomas.

The prominent signal void within the aqueduct and the marked proximal and distal extent of this signal void are due to hyperdynamic CSF flow and turbulence. The high-flow state accompanies communicating hydrocephalus with intact cerebral perfusion. The thin rim of periventricular high intensity represents transependymal resorption of CSF. An incidental cavum septum pellucidum is noted.

In the trauma patient, communicating hydrocephalus usually develops by the end of the second posttraumatic week. Approximately 5% of patients with severe head trauma will develop either obstructive or communicating hydrocephalus.

Reference

1. Bradley WG. Hydrocephalus and atrophy. In: Bradley WG, Stark DD, eds. *Magnetic resonance imaging.* St. Louis: CV Mosby Company, 1988.

Submitted by: Louis M. Teresi, M.D., Stephen J. Davis, M.D., and Mark Ziemba, M.D., Huntington Medical Research Institutes, Pasadena, California; William G. Bradley, Jr., M.D., Ph.D., Senior Editor.

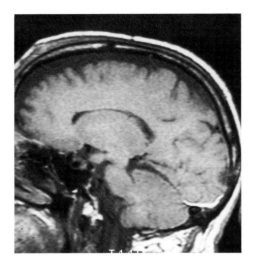

FIG. 47A. SE 600/20.

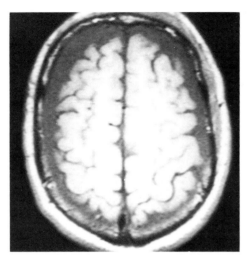

FIG. 47B. SE 800/20.

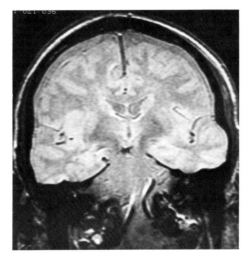

FIG. 47C. SE 2,800/30.

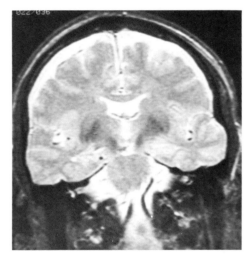

FIG. 47D. SE 2,800/70.

Clinical History

A 63-year-old physician initially hospitalized for motor vehicle accident and loss of consciousness (20 minutes). At that time, headache was the only finding. Now, the patient has returned two weeks after discharge from an outside hospital with increasing headache, nausea, vomiting, and dehydration.

Findings

Bilateral extra-axial collections are seen, the signal intensity of which is very much like that of normal cerebrospinal fluid (CSF). Note the relative lack of sulcal compression or other signs of mass effect on the brain. The slightly higher signal intensity of the extra-axial collections on the T1-weighted (Figs. 47A and B) and first echo, long TR (Fig. 47C) images is attributable to the CSF pulsation-induced signal loss within the ventricular system when compared with the subdural space. The second echo image (Fig. 47D) does not distinguish benign CSF from other fluid collections.

Incidentally noted, on the sagittal image (Fig. 47A) is a curvilinear high signal intensity collection underlying the left occipital pole consistent with a small amount of subarachnoid hemorrhage collecting in this dependent brain region.

Diagnosis

Posttraumatic CSF hygromas.

Discussion

The delayed appearance of extra-axial fluid following head trauma can be due to unrecognized subdural hematoma and rebleeding or to the slow egress of CSF from the arachnoid space into the subdural space due to arachnoid membrane tear. The latter is the most likely etiology for the collections noted here. The prognosis in such cases is much more benign than in true subdural bleeds. These collections tend to appear much later than traumatic subdural hematomas and resolve spontaneously over time with expectant management.

Magnetic resonance scanning can be quite useful in delineating the difference between CSF hygromas and chronic subdural hematomas based on the signal intensity of the fluid encountered. Computed tomography scans demonstrate both chronic subdural hematomas and hygromas as low-density collections. Magnetic resonance scanning can differentiate the bloody nature of the chronic hygroma on the basis of marked elevation of signal intensity on the first echo of the long TR sequence, as well as the T1-weighted sequences when the hematoma is relatively recent.

References

1. Kao S. Sedimentation level in chronic subdural hematoma visible on computerized tomography. *J Neurosurg* 1983;58:246–251.
2. Markwalder M. Chronic subdural hematomas: a review. *J Neurosurg* 1981;54:637–645.
3. Masuzawa O. Computed tomographic evolution of posttraumatic subdural hygromas in young adults. *Neuroradiology* 1984;26:245–248.
4. Gomori J, et al. Variable appearance of subacute intracranial hematomas on high field spin-echo MR. *AJNR* 1987;8:1019–1026.
5. Hayman A, et al. Pathophysiology of acute intracerebral and subarachnoid hemorrhage: applications to MR imaging. *AJNR* 1989;10:457–461.
6. Moon K, et al. Nuclear magnetic resonance imaging of CT —isodense subdural hematomas. *AJNR* 1984;5:319–322.
7. Seelig S, et al. Traumatic acute subdural hematoma. *N Engl J Med* 1981;304:1511–1518.

Submitted by: Michael Brant-Zawadzki, M.D., Senior Editor.

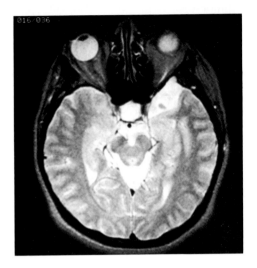 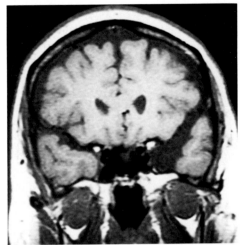

FIG. 48A. SE 2,800/70.   FIG. 48B. SE 600/20.

Clinical History

A 41-year-old woman with headaches.

Findings

A fluid collection is apparent anterior to the left temporal pole. The signal intensity is identical to that of cerebrospinal fluid (CSF). The CSF signal is the same within the arachnoid cyst as within the CSF-filled arachnoid pouch above the compressed pituitary gland ("partially empty sella"). Note the enlarged middle fossa, with thinning and scalping of the greater sphenoid wing shown on the axial T2-weighted view (Fig. 48A), as well as elevation of the lesser sphenoid wing shown on the T1-weighted coronal view (Fig. 48B).

Diagnosis

Left middle fossa arachnoid cyst.

Discussion

Cerebrospinal fluid collections in this location can result from atrophy of the temporal lobe, be it due to prior trauma (a typical location for that entity) or ischemia. The differentiation from an arachnoid cyst may be difficult. The latter entity represents a duplication of the arachnoid membrane, resulting in cyst development. The arachnoid cyst tends to produce enlargement of the middle fossa due to progressive remodeling of the bony confines, as in this case. These cysts generally do not communicate with the arachnoid space; a CT scan with intrathecal dye injection can be done to verify the lack of communication. Occasionally, such cysts will fill through a ball-valve mechanism.

Other entities, such as loculated subdural or epidural hematomas, can exist here, but the signal intensity of these collections would be higher than that of CSF on the T1-weighted image as well as on the 1st echo of the T2-weighted sequence.

References

1. Wilkins R, et al. Benign intraparenchymal brain cysts without an epithelial lining. *J Neurosurg* 1988;86:378–382.
2. Wiener S, et al. MR imaging of intracranial arachnoid cysts. *J Comput Assist Tomogr* 1987;11:236–241.
3. Kjos B, et al. Cystic intracranial lesions: magnetic resonance imaging. *Radiology* 1985;155:363–369.

Submitted by: Michael Brant-Zawadzki, M.D., Senior Editor.

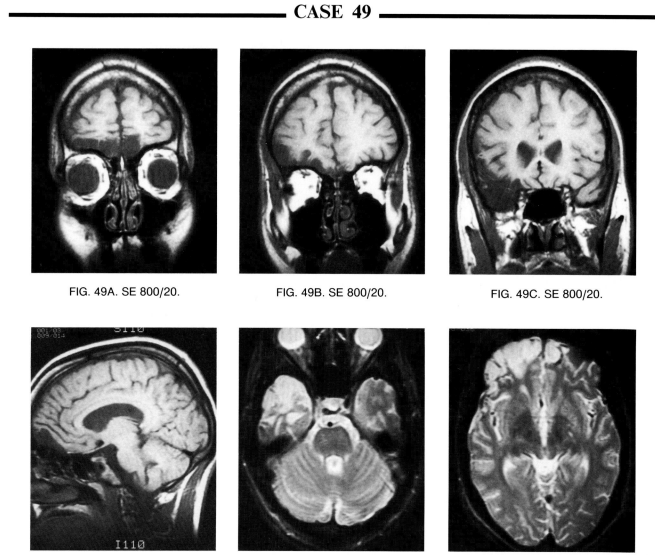

FIG. 49A. SE 800/20.   FIG. 49B. SE 800/20.   FIG. 49C. SE 800/20.

FIG. 49D. SE 600/20.   FIG. 49E. SE 2,800/80.   FIG. 49F. SE 2,800/80.

Clinical History

A 20-year-old man with seizures following head trauma.

Findings

The coronal T1-weighted (Figs. 49A–C), T1-weighted sagittal (Fig. 49D), and T2-weighted axial (Figs. 49E and F) images depict cystic changes in the subfrontal region of both hemispheres, greater on the right and extending into the temporal region. There is associated atrophy of the temporal gyri and enlargement of the right temporal horn. Note that the signal intensity is equal in the cystic collections to that of cerebrospinal fluid (CSF).

Diagnosis

Posttraumatic encephalomalacia and atrophy.

Discussion

This is the prototypical appearance of posttraumatic brain atrophy in the classic locations at the base of the skull where the inner irregularities of the calvarium are the greatest and scrape and contuse the brain during impact injury where the calverium is displaced relative to the brain. The end result of such contusion is brain atrophy, resulting in the multicystic appearance in the floor of the anterior and middle fossa as shown here. The intensity of the fluid being identical to CSF, the compensatory enlargement of the temporal horn, and the deformity of the temporal lobe all testify to old trauma as the primary etiology here.

Reference

1. Willberger JE, Deeb Z, Rothfus W. Magnetic resonance imaging in cases of severe head injury. *Neurosurgery* 1987;20:571–576.

Submitted by: Michael Brant-Zawadzki, M.D., Senior Editor.

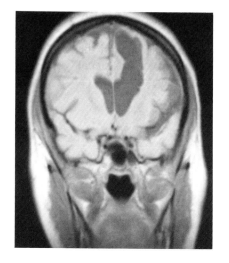

FIG. 51A. SE 1,000/30.

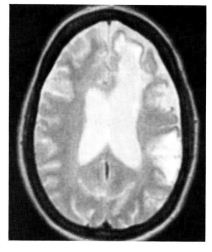

FIG. 51B. SE 3,000/80.

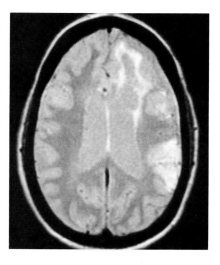

FIG. 51C. SE 3,000/40.

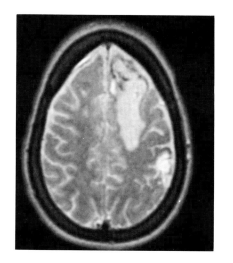

FIG. 51D. SE 3,000/80.

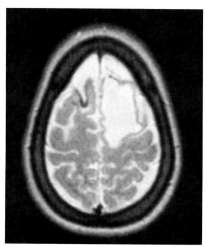

FIG. 51E. SE 3,000/80.

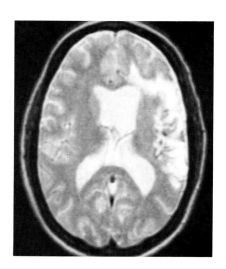

FIG. 51F. SE 3,000/80.

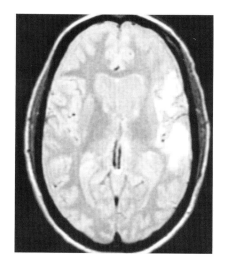

FIG. 51G. SE 3,000/40.

Clinical History

A 39-year-old woman, 18 months following left-sided head injury with recent blurred vision.

Findings

Axial 5 mm T2-W (SE 3,000/40 and 80) and coronal 10 mm T1-W (1,000/30) images are presented. There is a large cerebrospinal fluid intensity cyst communicating with the anterior aspect of the left lateral ventricle within the left frontal lobe (Figs. 51A and B). Surrounding the cyst is a thin rim of increased signal on the T2-weighted images, representing gliosis (Fig. 51C). There is gyriform decreased signal intensity within the anterior cyst wall on the T2-weighted images (Fig. 51D) with evidence of T2 shortening, the signal becoming progressively decreased in intensity with longer TE. There are similar separate, more prominent gyriform bands of T2 shortening involving the anterior cortex of the right frontal lobe (Fig. 51E) and the left insular cortex (Fig. 51F), both of these regions also showing focal cortical atrophy.

Multiple focal areas of increased signal intensity are present in the cortex of the left temporal lobe, left posterior frontal operculum, left insular cortex, and underlying extreme and external capsules (Fig. 51G). There is dilatation of the adjacent cerebral sulci and sylvian fissure, indicating focal brain atrophy in this region.

Diagnosis

Posttraumatic left frontal porencephalic cyst with severe atrophy of the left posterofrontal, temporal, and parietal lobes; evidence of previous cortical hemorrhage with hemosiderin deposition involving the anterior aspect of the left frontal porencephalic cyst, the anterior aspect of a focally atrophic right frontal lobe, and within the left insular cortex; and multifocal cortical atrophy involving the right frontal, left frontal, left temporal, and insular cortices.

Discussion

Porencephaly is a region of cavitation caused by brain necrosis, secondary to a variety of factors, either developmental or acquired. In adults, it is almost always acquired and usually due to trauma, hemorrhage, infection, surgery, or a vasco-occlusive process.

The cavity is often lined with ependymal cells and may be isolated or communicate with the ventricles or subarachnoid space. The rim of T2 shortening seen anteriorly in this cyst represents hemosiderin deposition, indicating that this cyst is likely to be posttraumatic in origin.

Similar hemosiderin deposition is noted in the right frontal lobe cortex overlying a focal area of atrophy and in the left insular cortex and residual temporal lobe. These lesions are all typical sequelae of posttraumatic hemorrhagic necrosis and posttraumatic atrophy of the brain.

Cortical hemosiderin deposition is also seen following hemorrhagic infarctions, although the bifrontal distribution and previous history of left-sided head trauma is against this diagnosis in this case.

Reference

1. Gentry LR, Godersky JC, Thompson B. MR imaging of head trauma: review of the distribution and radiopathological features of traumatic lesion. *AJNR* 1988;9:101–110.

Submitted by: Stephen J. Davis, M.D. and Louis M. Teresi, M.D., Huntington Medical Research Institutes, Pasadena, California; William G. Bradley, Jr., M.D., Ph.D., Senior Editor.

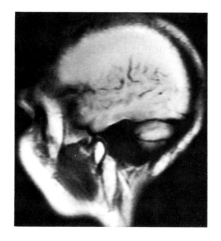 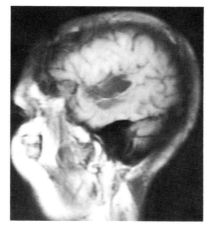 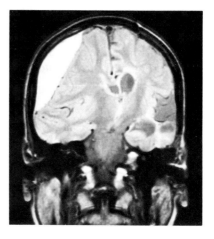

FIG. 53A. SE 800/20.   FIG. 53B. SE 800/20.   FIG. 53C. SE 2,500/20.

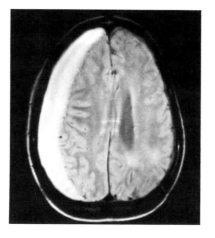 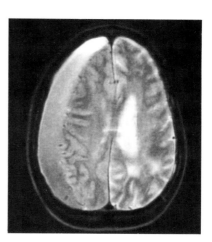

FIG. 53D. SE 2,500/20.   FIG. 53E. SE 2,500/70.

Clinical History

A 42-year-old woman who, in the emergency room, had sudden onset of severe headache, signs of increased intracranial pressure, and left hemiparesis.

Findings

A large subdural collection of fluid is seen over the right convexity. This has high-intensity signal characteristics on T1 weighting (Figs. 53A and B) as well as the first echo of the T2-weighted images (Figs. 53C and D). Marked midline shift is apparent: the coronal images show early uncal herniation on the right as well as entrapment at the left lateral ventricle. Incidentally noted is a focal cystic encephalomalacia of the left temporal lobe (Figs. 53B and C) (history of severe head trauma many years prior to the current presentation was elicited). Note that the signal intensity of the collection on the second echo image (Fig. 53E) fades, particularly in the dependent portion of the collection, the prefrontal component maintaining high signal intensity.

Diagnosis

Acute subdural hematoma, spontaneous, and old posttraumatic cystic encephalomalacia, left temporal lobe.

Discussion

Acute subdural hematomas can occur with significant head trauma. Also, relatively minor head trauma, which the patient may disregard, can produce subdural hematomas in patients with prior small chronic subdural collections or with relative atrophy (separation of the brain away from the inner table). Spontaneous bleeding into this increased extra-axial space can occur with grave consequences, as in this case. The signal intensity of the subdural collection reflects the nature of the fluid. Fresh blood containing red cells and intact oxyhemoglobin tends to appear relatively isointense. Once the oxyhemoglobin forms, the signal intensity diminishes due to magnetic susceptibility effects. Hematocrit, clot formation, and retraction, as well as the field strength of the instrument used, all play a role in the signal intensities seen.

In this case, the preferential loss of signal intensity on the second echo in the dependent portion of the collection, with preservation of high signal in the supernatant, suggests a large cellular component with the "hematocrit effect" (cells settling to the lower portion of the collection). Some cell lysis has already occurred, as shown by the high signal intensity on the T1-weighted images and in the supernatant produced by the methemoglobin component in solution.

References

1. Kao S. Sedimentation level in chronic subdural hematoma visible on computerized tomography. *J Neurosurg* 1983; 58:246–251.
2. Markwalder M. Chronic subdural hematomas: a review. *J Neurosurg* 1981;54:637–645.
3. Masuzawa O. Computed tomographic evolution of posttraumatic subdural hygromas in young adults. *Neuroradiology* 1984;26:245–248.
4. Gomori J, et al. Variable appearances of subacute intracranial hematomas on high field spin-echo MR. *AJNR* 1987;8:1019–1026.
5. Hayman A, et al. Pathophysiology of acute intracerebral and subarachnoid hemorrhage: applications to MR imaging. *AJNR* 1989;10:457–461.
6. Moon K, et al. Nuclear magnetic resonance imaging of CT —isodense subdural hematomas. *AJNR* 1984;5:319–322.

Submitted by: Michael Brant-Zawadzki, M.D., Senior Editor.

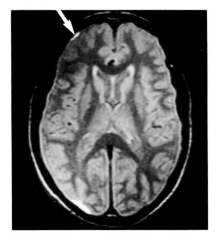
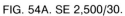
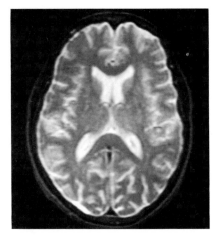

FIG. 54A. SE 2,500/30.　　　　　FIG. 54B. SE 2,500/80.

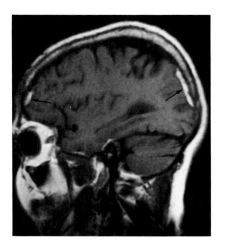

FIG. 54C. SE 600/20.

Clinical History

A 72-year-old woman who has suffered multiple falls and now complains of persistent headache.

Findings

Axial T2-W (SE 2,500/30 and 80) and sagittal T1-W (SE 600/20) images are provided for review. The axial SE 2,500/30 image shows two foci of increased signal intensity: one anterior to the right frontal lobe and the other posterior to the right occipital lobe (Fig. 54A). Both of these areas are much less conspicuous on the more T2-W SE 2,500/80 sequence, as they are not well contrasted against high-intensity surrounding cerebrospinal fluid (Fig. 54B). The sagittal T1-weighted images show that both areas obtain a high signal intensity compared with underlying brain (Fig. 54C, *arrows*).

Diagnosis

Late subacute subdural hematomas.

Discussion

During the late subacute stage (CT isodense), the red blood cells lyse and deoxyhemoglobin becomes oxidized to methemoglobin. These effects shorten T1 and lengthen T2, both of which will increase the intensity on T1- and T2-weighted images.

Reference

1. Fobben E, Grossman RI, Atlas SW, et al. MR characteristic of subdural hematomas and hygromas at 1.5T. *AJNR* 1989;10:687–693.

Submitted by: Louis M. Teresi, M.D., Stephen J. Davis, M.D., and Mark Ziemba, M.D., Huntington Medical Research Institutes, Pasadena, California; William G. Bradley, Jr., M.D., Ph.D., Senior Editor.

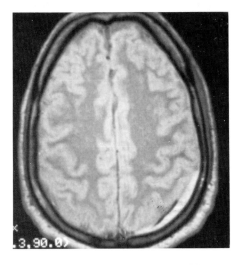

FIG. 55A. SE 3,000/25 and 80.

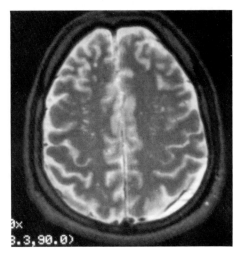

FIG. 55B. SE 3,000/80.

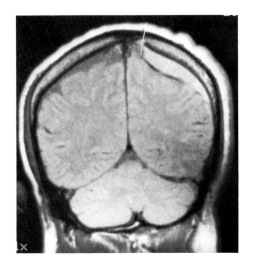

FIG. 55C. SE 700/30.

Clinical History

A 60-year-old man complaining of headaches two weeks following an auto accident.

Findings

The T2-weighted axial examination shows that there is an extra-axial fluid collection over the left parietal lobe (Figs. 55A and B). The first echo shows that the fluid collection has a signal intensity that is substantially higher than that of cerebrospinal fluid (CSF); the second echo shows that the intensity of the fluid collection has increased further, approximating that of CSF. There is no evidence of significant mass effect on underlying brain. The coronal T1-weighted image shows that the fluid collection is much brighter than CSF and is slightly brighter than underlying brain (Fig. 55C).

Diagnosis

Subacute subdural hematoma.

Discussion

Subdural hematomas have four distinct stages of evolution: hyperacute, acute, subacute, and chronic. During the subacute stage, the red blood cells lyse, and deoxyhemoglobin becomes oxidized to methemoglobin. If they occur synchronously, these effects tend to shorten the T1 and lengthen the T2, both of which will increase the intensity on either T1- or T2-weighted images.

The definition of a chronic subdural hematoma depends on whether the determination is being made clinically, by CT hypointensity, or by MR. Continued oxidative denaturization of methomoglobin forms hemichromes, which are low-spin, nonparamagnetic compounds. The T1 of such compounds is greater than that of paramagnetic methemoglobin; thus, chronic subdural hematomas are less intense than subacute subdural hematomas, particularly on T1-weighted images. Chronic subdural hematomas are still more intense than CSF, however, because of their higher protein concentration.

Reference

1. Fobben JA, Grossman RI, Atlas SW, et al. MR characteristics of subdural hematomas and hygromas at 1.5 T. *AJR* 1989;153:589–595.

Submitted by: Louis M. Teresi, M.D., Stephen J. Davis, M.D., and Mark Ziemba, M.D., Huntington Medical Research Institutes, Pasadena, California; William G. Bradley, Jr., M.D., Ph.D., Senior Editor.

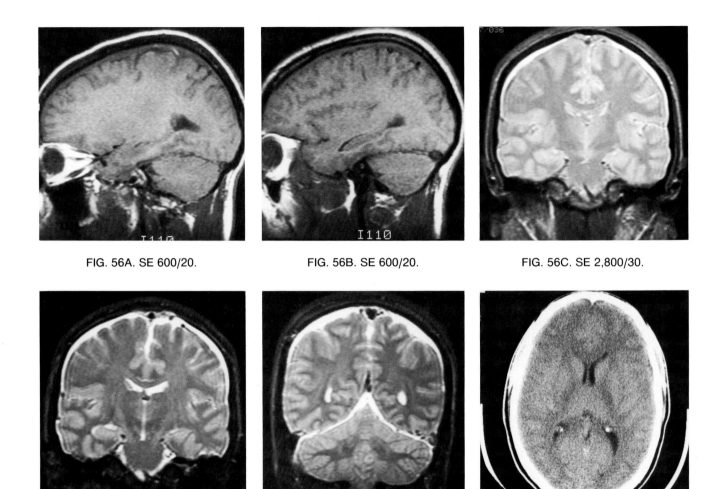

FIG. 56A. SE 600/20.

FIG. 56B. SE 600/20.

FIG. 56C. SE 2,800/30.

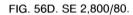

FIG. 56D. SE 2,800/80.

FIG. 56E. SE 2,800/80.

FIG. 56F. CT.

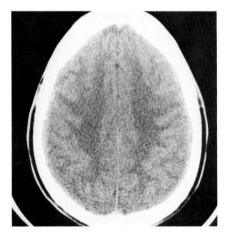

FIG. 56G. CT.

Clinical History

A 34-year-old man with a month-long history of headaches. Minor head trauma (a bar hit the patient's face during bench presses while weight lifting) was suffered at about the time of headache onset.

Findings

Curvilinear collections are present in the subdural space both on the T1-weighted sagittal (Figs. 56A and B) and the T2-weighted dual-echo (Figs. 56C–E) sequences. The signal intensity of the collection is isointense with gray matter on the T1-weighted image, clearly higher in signal than normal cerebrospinal fluid (CSF). This is corroborated by the two echoes of the dual-echo sequence. Of interest, the CT scan fails to delineate the collections (Figs. 56F and G).

Diagnosis

Subacute subdural hematoma.

Discussion

Subdural hematomas may be difficult to detect with CT, particularly when the collections are small, as the beam-hardening artifact of the calvarium makes contrast distinction of subacute collections difficult. Even larger subdural collections, particularly when isodense, can be difficult to diagnose on CT. Magnetic resonance scanning can readily detect these due to the optimal contrast differentiation between brain, fluid, and bone. Detection of even small subdural hematomas is important, as these collections may produce significant symptomatology even when relatively thin, due to the fact that the surface area over the convexity is quite large and the overall pressure-volume relationship may be altered by even relatively small collections. Also, the presence of subdural hematoma predisposes to a secondary bleed. This is due to the fact that bridging veins are stretched between the inner table and the cortex; minor trauma can produce sufficient shear to disrupt these. Also, the collections incite a capillary proliferation on the inner membrane of the dura and contain an anti-coagulant, both of these factors combining to produce a more friable capillary bed and repeated bleeding.

The appearance of subdural blood on MR can vary, depending on the overall hematocrit, the field strength of the instrument used, the status of the hemoglobin molecule, and the presence of clot.

Differential diagnosis for subdural collections include dural spread of tumor (more likely to be irregular in its appearance), subdural empyema (most often in the setting of an acutely ill patient), and thickened, reactive dura (seen in patients with prior bleeding, surgery, or intrathecal therapy). The use of intravenous paramagnetic contrast can help in distinguishing subdural tumor or post-inflammatory dural thickening from frank fluid collections, as would be seen with acute or subacute subdural hematoma.

Occasionally, subdural collections of CSF can occur after trauma. These are thought to be due to tears of the arachnoid membrane and progressive ball-valve type of subdural accumulation of benign CSF. These generally appear on a delayed basis and resolve without the need for surgery. Such collections would have signal intensity identical with that of CSF on MR.

References

1. Moon K, et al. Nuclear magnetic resonance imaging of CT —isodense subdural hematomas. *AJNR* 1984;5:319–322.
2. Gomori J, et al. Variable appearances of subacute intracranial hematomas on high field spin-echo MR. *AJNR* 1987;8:1019–1026.
3. Hayman A, et al. Pathophysiology of acute intracerebral and subarachnoid hemorrhage: applications to MR imaging. *AJNR* 1989;10:457–461.
4. Seelig S, et al. Traumatic acute subdural hematoma. *N Engl J Med* 1981;304:1511–1518.

Submitted by: Michael Brant-Zawadzki, M.D., Senior Editor.

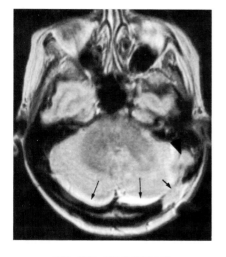

FIG. 57A. SE 3,000/40.

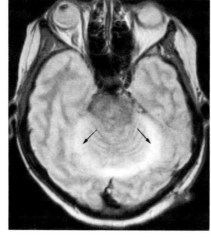

FIG. 57B. SE 3,000/40.

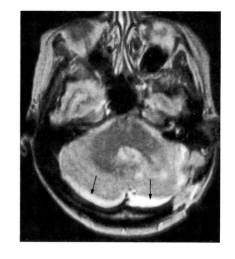

FIG. 57C. SE 3,000/80.

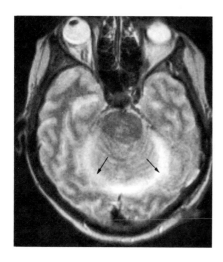

FIG. 57D. SE 3,000/80.

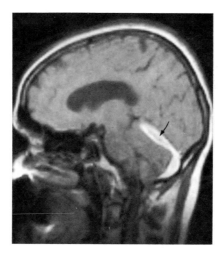

FIG. 57E. SE 500/40.

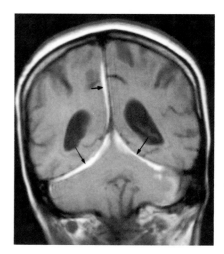

FIG. 57F. SE 500/30.

Clinical History

A 60-year-old woman, two weeks after resection of posterior fossa meningioma, who is complaining of headache.

Findings

Axial T2-W (SE 3,000/40 and 80), coronal T1-W (SE 500/30), and sagittal T1-W (SE 500/40) images are provided for review. The axial SE 3,000/40 images reveal the postoperative defect (Fig. 57A, *short arrow*) and residual meningioma in the left posterior fossa (Fig. 57A, *arrowhead*). High-intensity material is seen posterior to the cerebellum bilaterally (Fig. 57A, *long arrows*). On more cephalad images, high intensity is also noted on both sides of the falx (Fig. 57B, *arrows*). Both the region posterior to the cerebellum and around the tentorium further increase in intensity on the SE 3,000/80 sequence (Figs. 57C and D, *arrows*). The sagittal T1-weighted image shows that the region posterior to the cerebellum is contiguous with that of the falx and is high intensity relative to brain (Fig. 57E, *arrow*). Coronal T1-weighted images show the high-intensity subdural tentorial collections (Fig. 57F, *long arrows*), as well as a high-intensity collection in the region of the falx (Fig. 57F, *short arrow*). Neither the falx nor the tentorial collections extend into underlying cortical sulci.

Diagnosis

Tentorial and falcine late subacute subdural hematomas.

Discussion

Late subacute subdural hematomas have lysed red blood cells and free methemoglobin. These effects shorten T1 and lengthen T2, both of which will increase the intensity on either T1- or T2-weighted images.

Tentorial subdural hematomas are uncommon and are seen more frequently in postoperative patients than in those with closed head trauma. They occur in approximately 0.01% of all head injuries (2). In the neonate, birth injury and traumatic delivery can disrupt the tentorium and veins that bridge from the cerebellum through the potential subdural space into the intradural sinuses, leading to subdural hematoma. Tentorial subdurals are distinguished from subarachnoid hemorrhage by noting that the blood products do not extend into underlying cortical sulci. Small tentorial subdurals may be missed on CT; however, the multiplanar imaging capabilities of MR facilitate their identification.

References

1. Fobben E, Grossman RI, Atlas SW, et al. MR characteristic of subdural hematomas and hygromas at 1.5T. *AJNR* 1989;10:687–693.
2. Bakay L, Glasauer FE, Alker GJ, eds. *Head injury.* Boston: Little, Brown, 1980;191–236.

Submitted by: Louis M. Teresi, M.D., Stephen J. Davis, M.D., and Mark Ziemba, M.D., Huntington Medical Research Institutes, Pasadena, California; William G. Bradley, Jr., M.D., Ph.D., Senior Editor.

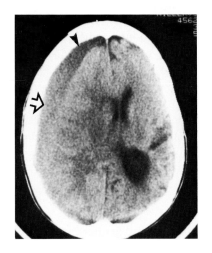

FIG. 58A. CT.

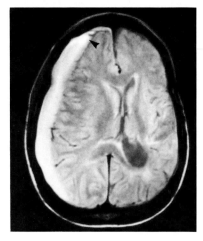

FIG. 58B. SE 2,500/20.

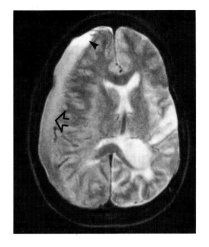

FIG. 58C. SE 2,500/70.

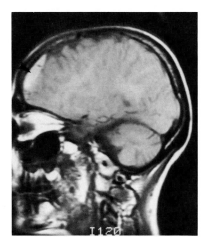

FIG. 58D. SE 800/20.

Clinical History

A 42-year-old woman seven days after a fall.

Findings

Axial T2-W (SE 2,500/20 and 70) and sagittal T1-W (SE 800/20) images are provided for review. An axial non-contrast CT is also provided and shows a large, mostly isodense subdural fluid collection on the right (Fig. 58A, *open arrow*). The anterior aspect of the subdural collection (Fig. 58A, *arrowhead*) is significantly less dense than the posterior aspect. Axial SE 2,500/20 MR images show the subdural as higher signal intensity than brain, with the most anterior aspect (Fig. 58B, *arrowhead*), being more intense than the more posterior portion. On the 2,500/70 axial image the anterior aspect of the subdural remains hyperintense (Fig. 58C, *arrowhead*), whereas the posterior aspect (Fig. 58C, *open arrow*) becomes significantly less intense, approaching that of underlying brain. The T1-weighted sagittal SE 800/20 image shows that the anterior aspect of the subdural is hyperintense (Fig. 58D, *arrowhead*).

Diagnosis

Subacute subdural hematoma.

Discussion

The dependent collection represents intact red blood cells containing methemoglobin. This appears bright on T1-weighted images and dark on T2-weighted images due to magnetic nonuniformity. The nondependent collection represents methemoglobin free in solution and is high signal on both T1- and T2-weighted images.

Reference

1. Fobben E, Grossman RI, Atlas SW, et al. MR characteristic of subdural hematomas and hygromas at 1.5T. *AJNR* 1989;10:687–693.

Submitted by: Louis M. Teresi, M.D., Stephen J. Davis, M.D., and Mark Ziemba, M.D., Huntington Medical Research Institutes, Pasadena, California; William G. Bradley, Jr., M.D., Ph.D., Senior Editor.

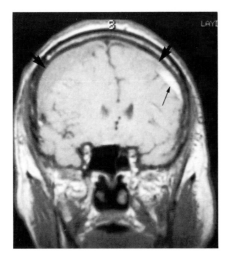

FIG. 59A. SE 750/30.

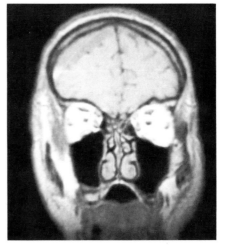

FIG. 59B. SE 750/30.

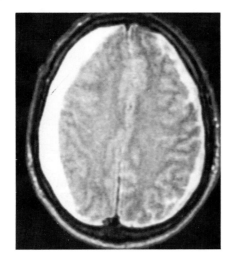

FIG. 59C. SE 3,000/80.

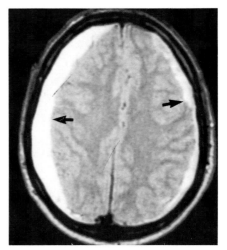

FIG. 59D. SE 3,000/40.

Clinical History

A 65-year-old man with a history of falling and dementia.

Findings

Axial T2-W (SE 3,000/40 and 80) and coronal T1-W (SE 750/30) images are provided for review. The coronal images show extra-axial fluid collections bilaterally (Fig. 59A, *large short arrows*) that are mostly slightly hypointense relative to brain; however, they do show a small amount of increased signal in the inferior portions of both collections (Figs. 59A and B, *long arrows*). The axial T2-weighted images show that both high- and low-signal regions on the T1-weighted study acquire high signal on both echoes (Fig. 59D, *arrows*).

Diagnosis

Chronic subdural hematomas with evidence of rehemorrhage.

Discussion

The MR characteristics of acute and subacute subdural hematomas are similar to those of intraparenchymal hemorrhage, whereas chronic subdural hematomas differ from parenchymal hematomas in several ways. As opposed to the typical chronic parenchymal hematoma, which is markedly hyperintense on T1-weighted images, a chronic subdural hematoma will usually be slightly hypointense to isointense relative to gray matter on T1-weighted images. This loss of the T1-shortening effect appears to result from a decrease in the concentration of free methemoglobin by dilution, absorption, and/or degradation. In addition, hemosiderin is infrequently present in chronic subdural hematomas. However, the marked hypointensity of hemosiderin on the T2-weighted images may be seen in thickened membranes in the subdural collection.

Rehemorrhage is a frequent phenomenon with subdural hematomas, and MR offers excellent visualization of this process. Because of the presence of a vascular membrane, subdural hematomas are prone to rehemorrhaging even without clinically evident trauma (1). Rehemorrhage has been estimated to occur at an average rate of 10% of the subdural hematoma's volume per day using radionuclide-tagged red blood cells. In these cases, MR demonstrates repeat hemorrhages with layering and dilution of deoxyhemoglobin or methemoglobin in known chronic collections.

References

1. Ito H, Yamamoto S, Komai T, et al. Role of local hyperfibrinolysis in the etiology of chronic subdural hematoma. *J Neurosurg* 1976;45:26–30.
2. Fobben E, Grossman RI, Atlas SW, et al. MR characteristic of subdural hematomas and hygromas at 1.5T. *AJNR* 1989;10:687–693.

Submitted by: Louis M. Teresi, M.D., Stephen J. Davis, M.D., and Mark Ziemba, M.D., Huntington Medical Research Institutes, Pasadena, California; William G. Bradley, Jr., M.D., Ph.D., Senior Editor.

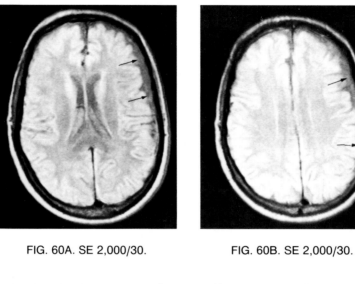

FIG. 60A. SE 2,000/30.   FIG. 60B. SE 2,000/30.

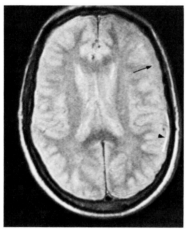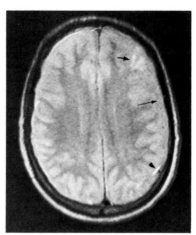

FIG. 60C. SE 2,000/60.   FIG. 60D. SE 2,000/60.

Clinical History

A 74-year-old man 48 hours after a fall in which he hit the right side of his head.

Findings

Axial T2-W (SE 2,000/30 and 60) images are provided for review. The axial SE 2,000/30 and SE 2,000/60 images show a crescent-shaped fluid collection on the left that is isointense to cerebrospinal fluid (CSF) on both sequences (Figs. 60A–D, *long arrows*). A small focus of increased signal intensity is seen in superficial cortical gyri in the left frontal lobe on the SE 2,000/60 images (Fig. 60D, *short arrow*), which is not appreciated on the SE 2,000/30 sequences. Linear high signal in the region of the fluid collection on the SE 2,000/60 images, not seen on the SE 2,000/30 sequences, represents even-echo rephasing in a superficial cortical vein (Figs. 60C and D, *arrowheads*).

Diagnosis

Subdural hygroma and posttraumatic cortical edema.

Discussion

Nonhemorrhagic acute subdural hygromas display signal intensities on T1- and T2-weighted sequences that follow CSF without evidence of hemorrhage (1). Fluid analysis demonstrates nonhemorrhagic, clear CSF. Such collections are presumably due to tears in the arachnoid membrane (4).

Cortical contusions comprise the second most common type of traumatic lesion found on MR (3). A cortical contusion involves only the superficial cortex with relative sparing of the underlying white matter. Cortical contusions are hemorrhagic approximately half the time, perhaps reflecting the extensive vascularity of the gray matter. The temporal lobe is the most common site (50%), followed by the frontal lobe (30%). Cortical contusions rarely resolve completely on MR, usually leaving regions of gliotic scarring.

References

1. Fobben E, Grossman RI, Atlas SW, et al. MR characteristic of subdural hematomas and hygromas at 1.5T. *AJNR* 1989;10:687–693.
2. Hesselink JR, Dowd CF, Healy M, et al. MR imaging of brain contusions: a comparative study with CT. *AJNR* 1988;9:269–278.
3. Gentry LR, Godersky JC, Thompson B. MR imaging of head trauma: review of the distribution and radiopathology features of traumatic lesions. *AJNR* 1988;9:101–110.
4. Hoff J, Bates E, Barnes B, et al. Traumatic hemosiderin hygroma. *J Trauma* 1973;13:870–876.

Submitted by: Louis M. Teresi, M.D. and Stephen J. Davis, M.D., Huntington Medical Research Institutes, Pasadena, California; William G. Bradley, Jr., M.D., Ph.D., Senior Editor.

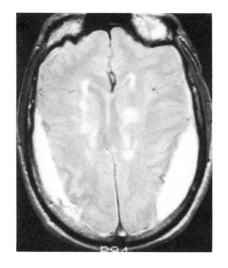

FIG. 61A. SE 3,300/30.

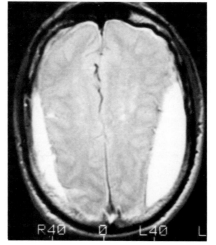

FIG. 61B. SE 3,300/30.

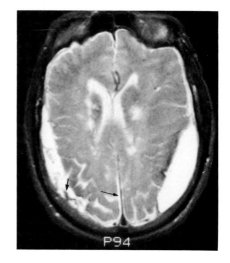

FIG. 61C. SE 3,300/80.

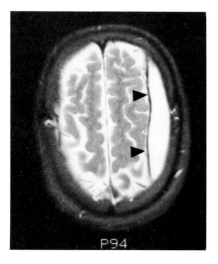

FIG. 61D. SE 3,300/80.

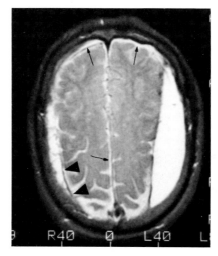

FIG. 61E. SE 3,300/80.

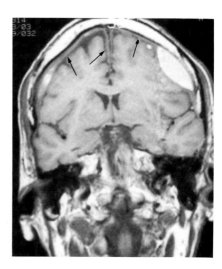

FIG. 61F. SE 600/20.

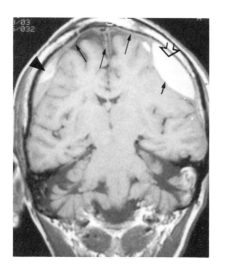

FIG. 61G. SE 600/20.

Clinical History

An 80-year-old man four weeks after evacuation of bilateral chronic subdural hematomas.

148

Findings

Axial T2-W (SE 3,300/30 and 80) and coronal T1-W (SE 600/20) images are provided for review. Axial and coronal images show a high-signal, lentiform-shaped extra-axial fluid collection over the left parietal lobe. On the T1-weighted coronal images, the medial aspect of the collection has a very high signal (Fig. 61G, *small, short arrow*), whereas the more peripheral portion has a somewhat lower signal intensity (Fig. 61G, *open arrow*). The collection has uniform high signal on the T2-weighted images. A low-signal interface separating the collection from underlying brain is noted on the T2-weighted axial images (Fig. 61D, *arrowheads*) but not on the T1-weighted images.

There is a second extra-axial collection on the right. Unlike the left-sided collection, it has a more crescentic, rather than biconvex, shape and has mixed signal intensity. The T1-weighted coronal images show that it is predominantly isointense, with an irregular high-signal region within it (Fig. 61G, *arrowhead*). Both the hyperintense and isointense regions become hyperintense on T2-weighted images. Scattered irregular low-signal regions are also seen in the right collection on the T2-weighted images only (Fig. 61C, *short arrow*). Like the left collection, the right collection also has a low-signal line between it and the underlying brain, seen best on the T2-weighted images (Fig. 61E, *arrowheads*).

Coronal T1-weighted images show intermediate signal material in the subdural space, which acquires a very high signal on the T2-weighted images, giving the appearance of uniform thickening of the subdural space (Figs. 61E–G, *long arrows*).

Diagnosis

Subacute-chronic subdural hematomas and meningeal fibrosis.

Discussion

The evolution of subacute to chronic subdural hematoma takes place after approximately three weeks. Whereas the subacute hematoma is hyperintense on T1-weighted images, a chronic subdural hematoma will usually be slightly hypointense to isointense relative to gray matter on T1-weighted images. Continued oxidative denaturation of methemoglobin forms hemichromes, which are low-spin, nonparamagnetic ferric compounds. The T1 of such compounds is greater than that of paramagnetic methemoglobin; therefore, chronic subdural hematomas are less intense than their subacute counterparts. In addition, there is infrequent presence of hemosiderin, manifested by hypointensity on T2-weighted images, in chronic subdural hematomas. The marked hypointensity of hemosiderin is seen in thickened membranes abutting the subdural collection. Chronic subdural hematomas usually remain more intense than cerebrospinal fluid due to their higher protein concentration.

The cause of meningeal fibrosis is unclear, but it probably represents a complication of one or more subdural hemorrhages resulting in a thick zone of fibrosis. Meningeal fibrosis occurs in association with chronic subdural hematomas in shunted and nonshunted patients. Pathologically, this entity is represented by a thick, fibrous membrane containing granulation tissue and increased vascularity. Meningeal fibrosis, therefore, has been observed to enhance with gadolinium-DTPA.

References

1. Bradley WG. Magnetic resonance imaging of the central nervous system. *Neurol Res* 1984;6:91–106.
2. Fobben E, Grossman RI, Atlas SW, et al. MR characteristic of subdural hematomas and hygromas at 1.5T. *AJNR* 1989;10:687–693.
3. Braun J, Borovich B, Guilburd JN, et al. Acute subdural hematoma mimicking epidural hematoma on CT. *AJNR* 1987;8:171.
4. Destian S, Heier LA, Zimmerman RD, et al. Differentiation between meningeal fibrosis and chronic subdural hematoma after ventricular shunting: value of enhanced CT and MR scans. *AJNR* 1989;10:1021–1026.

Submitted by: Louis M. Teresi, M.D. and Stephen J. Davis, M.D., Huntington Medical Research Institutes, Pasadena, California; William G. Bradley, Jr., M.D., Ph.D., Senior Editor.

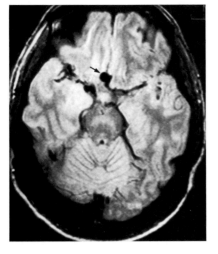

FIG. 62A. SE 2,500/30.

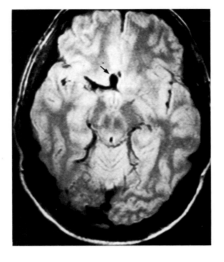

FIG. 62B. SE 2,500/30.

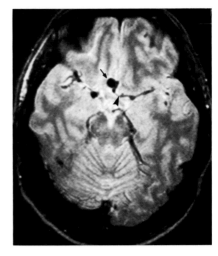

FIG. 62C. SE 2,500/60.

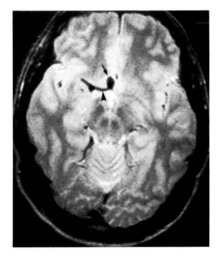

FIG. 62D. SE 2,500/60.

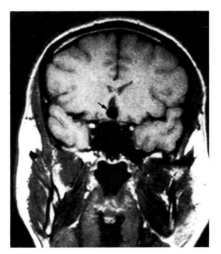

FIG. 62E. SE 600/30.

Clinical History

A 43-year-old man with headache.

Findings

Axial T2-W (SE 2,500/30 and 60) and coronal T1-W (SE 600/30) images are provided for review. The axial SE 2,500/30 and SE 2,500/60 images and coronal SE 600/30 image shows a rounded area with flow void in the region of the anterior communicating artery (Figs. 62A–E, *arrows*). Clear communication is noted between this flow-void structure and the A1 segments of the anterior cerebral arteries (Figs. 62C and D, *arrowheads*).

Diagnosis

Anterior communicating artery aneurysm.

Discussion

An aneurysm is a focal enlargement of an artery and may be saccular or fusiform. Aneurysms are classified as congenital, atherosclerotic, mycotic, or dissecting. The most common type is the congenital or berry aneurysm, thought to be a defect in the tunica media. The incidence in the general population is approximately 3%. Ninety-five percent of aneurysms involve the anterior circulation. In the anterior circulation, the most common location involves the origin of the anterior communicating artery (30%) followed by middle cerebral artery (25%) and posterior communicating artery (20%). Other sites in the anterior circulation are at the origin of the ophthalmic artery and the anterior choroidal artery. In the vertebral-basilar system, the most common site is the tip of the basilar artery, whereas other rare sites include origins of the posterior inferior cerebral artery. In approximately 20% of patients, more than one aneurysm can be demonstrated angiographically. The majority of the aneurysms detected on angiography following a subarachnoid hemorrhage are less than 1 cm in diameter. The large (1–2.5 cm) and giant (greater than 2.5 cm) aneurysms usually do not present with subarachnoid hemorrhage. They are most often associated with neurologic findings, due to either localized mass effect and pressure on the adjacent brain and cranial nerves or to thromoembolic phenomena, secondary to the turbulent flow within the aneurysm.

Magnetic resonance imaging has several advantages over CT in demonstrating the presence of an aneurysm, whether the patient has had subarachnoid hemorrhage or has neurologic findings secondary to the focal mass effect. Although flowing blood has a variable appearance depending on the direction and velocity of flow, in general, rapidly flowing blood has a dark appearance, a "signal void," both on T1- and T2-weighted images. The absence of signal is due to the excited protons leaving the selected section prior to emitting a spin-echo signal, as well as due to turbulence, and dephasing. High signal can also be seen in an aneurysm, particularly in larger aneurysms that have sluggish or stagnant flow within the lumen. High signal due to sluggish flow is most pronounced on long TE images.

Because of its inherent sensitivity to flow and products of hemorrhage, MRI, unlike CT, can visualize vascular structures without a contrast agent. Small aneurysms (less than 5 mm in diameter) can be missed, especially if they are not located completely in the voxel. However, if one uses thin contiguous slice acquisition, most aneurysms can be detected by MRI due to the high intrinsic contrast between flowing blood and brain.

References

1. Bradley WG. Flow phenomena. In: Stark DD, Bradley WG, eds. *Magnetic resonance imaging.* St. Louis: CV Mosby, 1988;108–137.
2. Olsen WL, Brant-Zawadzki M, Hodes J, et al. Giant intracranial aneurysms: MR imaging. *Radiology* 1987;163:431.
3. Atlas SW, Grossman RI, Goldberg HI, et al. Partially thrombosed giant intracranial aneurysms: correlation of MRI and pathological findings. *Radiology* 1987;162:111–114.

Submitted by: Louis M. Teresi, M.D. and Stephen J. Davis, M.D., Huntington Medical Research Institutes, Pasadena, California; William G. Bradley, Jr., M.D., Ph.D., Senior Editor.

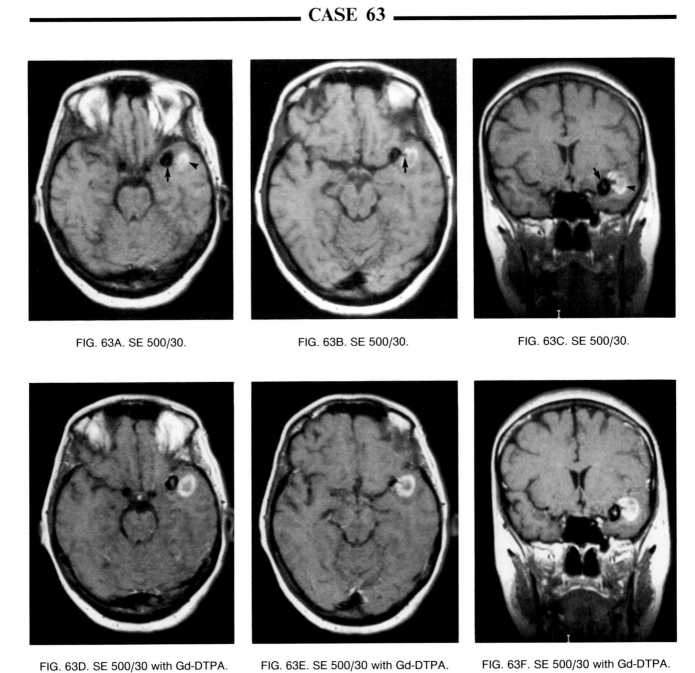

FIG. 63A. SE 500/30.

FIG. 63B. SE 500/30.

FIG. 63C. SE 500/30.

FIG. 63D. SE 500/30 with Gd-DTPA.

FIG. 63E. SE 500/30 with Gd-DTPA.

FIG. 63F. SE 500/30 with Gd-DTPA.

Clinical History

Two weeks prior to scanning, this 40-year-old woman developed a sudden severe occipital headache, followed three days later by an episode of sudden loss of consciousness.

Findings

T1-weighted images were obtained both before (Figs. 63A–C) and after (Figs. 63D–F) gadolinium-DTPA. There is a 1.5 cm diameter oval signal void immediately inferior to the left middle cerebral artery within the sylvian fissure (Figs. 63A and B, *arrow*). The center of the signal void region has a smaller area of intermediate signal intensity. Adjacent to this, within the left temporal lobe, is a 2 cm diameter rounded lesion with a high-intensity rim, an isointense center, and mild mass effect (Figs. 63A and C, *arrowhead*). A 3 mm diameter linear signal void passes between the two lesions superiorly (Fig. 63B, *arrow*).

Following gadolinium administration (Figs. 63D–F), there is a thin rim of contrast enhancement surrounding the signal void lesion and a slightly thicker rim of enhancement surrounding the adjacent high-intensity mass. The center of the signal void lesion also increases in intensity.

Diagnosis

Large middle cerebral aneurysm with adjacent subacute temporal lobe hematoma.

Discussion

The findings are typical of an aneurysm that has bled into the adjacent parenchyma. The signal void in the periphery of the aneurysm lumen represents signal loss, which is due to high velocity, turbulence, and dephasing. The center of the lumen has very sluggish flow; thus, the intermediate signal on precontrast images and increased signal on post-contrast images. This was confirmed by angiography. From the MR image alone, calcification, air, or extreme T2 shortening from paramagnetic substances such as hemosiderin would look alike. The small linear signal void entering the adjacent subacute hematoma is likely to represent the bleeding site.

The adjacent temporal lobe hematoma has the classic appearance of subacute hemorrhage with T1 shortening, shown on the pre-contrast images, due to methemoglobin. Although MR imaging cannot be used to exclude the presence of a small aneurysm, it may be useful in identifying the site of bleeding in a patient with known multiple aneurysms by the identification of subacute hemorrhage adjacent to it.

Giant aneurysms can be accurately diagnosed using MR imaging. These lesions are larger than 2.5 cm in size, occur most frequently in middle-aged women, and usually present as mass lesions, although subarachnoid hemorrhage does occur. They present with a "layered" appearance due to a flow void within the residual lumen and layers of mixed signal intensity representing various stages of mural thrombus. There is usually high-signal methemoglobin within this lamination.

References

1. Atlas SW, Grossman RI, Goldberg HI, et al. Partially thrombosed giant intracranial aneurysms: correlation of MR and pathological findings. *Radiology* 1987;162:111–114.
2. Hackney DB, Lesnick JE, Zimmerman RA, et al. Identification of bleeding site in subarachnoid hemorrhage with multiple intracranial aneurysms. *J Comput Assist Tomogr* 1986;10:878–880.

Submitted by: Stephen J. Davis, M.D., Louis M. Teresi, M.D., and Mark Ziemba, M.D., Huntington Medical Research Institutes, Pasadena, California: William G. Bradley, Jr., M.D., Ph.D., Senior Editor.

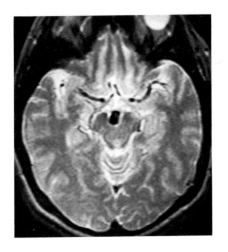 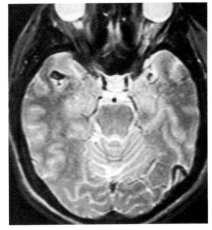

FIG. 64A. SE 2,800/80.   FIG. 64B. SE 2,800/80.

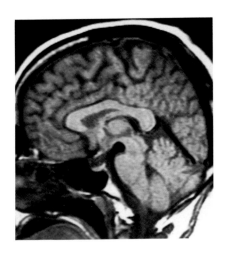 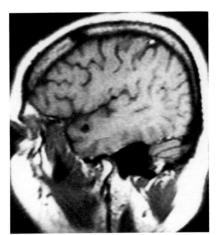

FIG. 64C. SE 600/20.   FIG. 64D. SE 600/20.

Clinical History

A 47-year-old woman with headaches.

Findings

The T2-weighted axial images (Figs. 64A and B) at the base of the brain depict a focus of very low signal in the interpeduncular cistern of the brainstem, which has a globular shape. A second, similar finding is present in the right temporal pole. The T1-weighted sequences (Figs. 64C and D) in the sagittal plane verify rounded, low-signal structures in both locations. Digital-subtraction angiography verifies aneurysms in both locations (Figs. 64E and F) but, in addition, shows a third aneurysm (Fig. 64G) in the left middle cerebral artery trifurcation not detected prospectively on the MRI study.

Diagnosis

Multiple aneurysms.

Discussion

The ability of MRI to depict flowing vessels due to time-of-flight effects as well as spin-phase changes is well known. This capability has been exploited for detection of intracranial aneurysms on both routine and specifically designed flow sequences. Aneurysms, in general, will appear as spherical or globular regions of signal void and may propagate phase artifacts in images with poor phase compensation. Clots within the aneurysm can be seen as regions of high signal, although flow effects may mimic such high-signal foci. Occasionally, turbulence and consequent dephasing due to pulsation of the basilar artery in the intrapeduncular cistern may mimic an aneu-

rysm of the basilar artery. Hence, the importance of confirming the finding on a second sequence, preferably in a different plane. The value of MR angiography in the detection of aneurysms is still being investigated. Nevertheless, the consensus of neuroradiologic opinion is that conventional angiography remains the "gold standard" for aneurysm screening, especially in the evaluation of patients with suspected subarachnoid hemorrhage. This case also demonstrates the difficulty routine MRI may have in detecting smaller aneurysms, such as the left middle cerebral artery aneurysm in this patient.

References

1. Worthington BS, Kein DM, Hawkes RC. NMR imaging in the recognition of giant intracranial aneurysms. *AJNR* 1983;4:835–836.
2. Olsen WL, Brant-Zawadzki M, Hodes J, et al. Giant intracranial aneurysms: MR imaging. *Radiology* 1987;163:431–435.
3. Burt TB. MR of CSF flow phenomenon mimicking basilar artery aneurysm. *AJNR* 1987;8:55–58.
4. Masaryk TJ, Modic MT, Ross JS, et al. Intracranial circulation: preliminary clinical results with three-dimensional MR angiography. *Radiology* 1989;171:793–799.

Submitted by: Michael Brant-Zawadzki, M.D., Senior Editor.

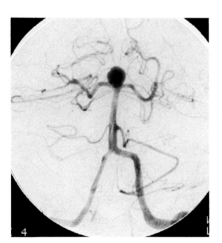

FIG. 64E. Angiogram.

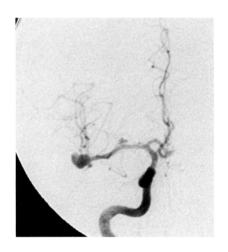

FIG. 64F. Angiogram.

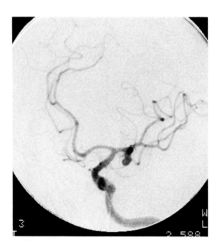

FIG. 64G. Angiogram.

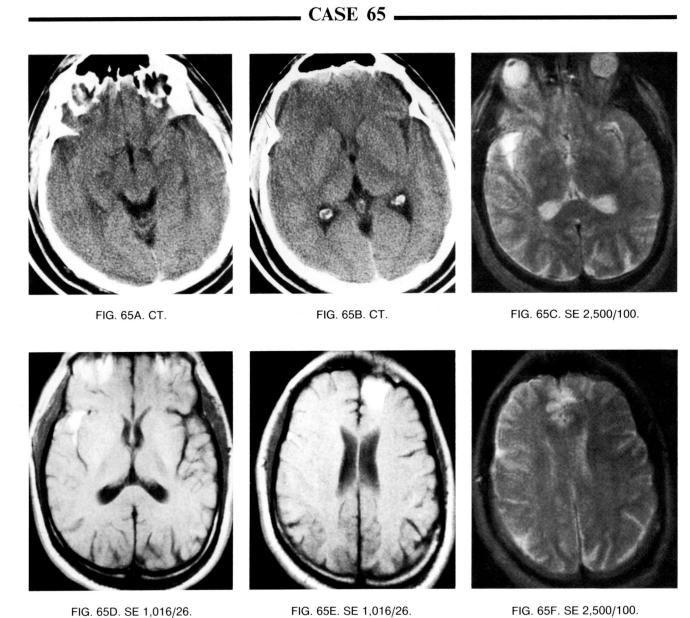

FIG. 65A. CT.

FIG. 65B. CT.

FIG. 65C. SE 2,500/100.

FIG. 65D. SE 1,016/26.

FIG. 65E. SE 1,016/26.

FIG. 65F. SE 2,500/100.

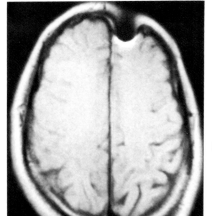

FIG. 65G. SE 1,016/26.

Clinical History

A 44-year-old man with sudden onset of left body weakness and altered mental status. A CT-scan was ordered to rule out infarct.

Findings

The CT scan (done without contrast) showed no abnormality except for asymmetry of the sylvian cisterns: note the absence of the right sylvian cistern (Figs. 65A and B). Because of this finding, an MRI scan was performed. This showed two abnormalities. The sylvian fissure reveals a collection with high signal intensity within it, both on T2- and T1-weighted axial images (Figs. 65C and D, respectively). At a higher level, a second high signal abnormality was noted in the left frontal pole (Fig. 65E), which was not corroborated on the T2-weighted image (Fig. 65F). Indeed, the T1-weighted axial image immediately below (Fig. 65G) shows a more artifactual appearance of the frontal calvarium. Scrutiny of the CT scan at the same level (Fig. 65H) reveals a punctate metallic foreign body in the scalp adjacent to the calvarium.

Because of the abnormalities in this sylvian fissure, which suggested clot, an angiogram was performed and revealed an aneurysm with evidence of spasm, the spasm having produced the syndrome responsible for the patient's presentation.

Diagnosis

Focal subarachnoid hemorrhage from right middle cerebral artery aneurysm, as well as ferromagnetic artifact suggesting hemorrhage elsewhere.

Discussion

Magnetic resonance imaging can be particularly useful in patients who present with sequelae of subarachnoid hemorrhage that went unnoticed. Because CT scanning can miss the presence of blood in the subarachnoid space following the denaturation of the blood proteins, it may take frank infarction of the brain to make the presence of subarachnoid hemorrhage-induced spasm known. The finding of clot on the MRI scan prompts the appropriate angiographic study.

Ferromagnetic artifact can simulate the presence of a hemorrhagic lesion on T1-weighted sequences. However, the distortion of the magnetic field produced can generally be discerned, as in this case (Fig. 65G). The clue to the lack of real hemorrhage was the absence of the "lesion" on the corresponding image (Fig. 65F) obtained with T2 weighing. Very small metallic foci can produce surprisingly large artifacts depending on their composition, as in this case.

References

1. Haacke EM, Bellon EM. Artifacts in magnetic resonance imaging. In: Stark DD, Bradley WG, eds. *Magnetic Resonance Imaging.* St. Louis: CV Mosby, 1988;138–158.
2. Satoh S, Kadoya S. Magnetic resonance imaging of subarachnoid hemorrhage. *Neuroradiology* 1988;30:361–366.

Submitted by: Michael Brant-Zawadzki, M.D., Senior Editor.

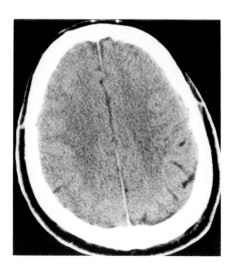

FIG. 65H. CT.

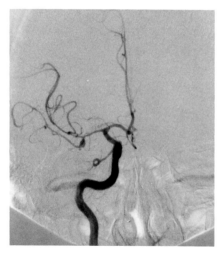

FIG. 65I. Angiogram.

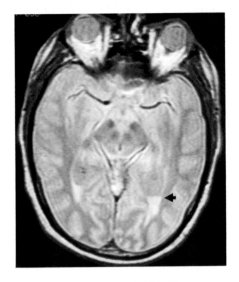

FIG. 66A. SE 2,800/30.

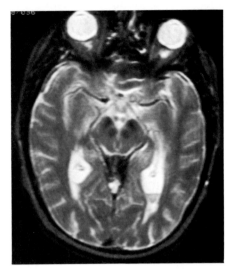

FIG. 66B. SE 2,800/90.

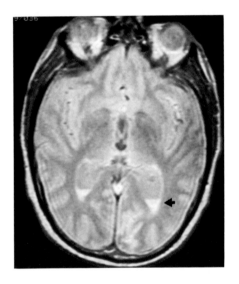

FIG. 66C. SE 2,800/30.

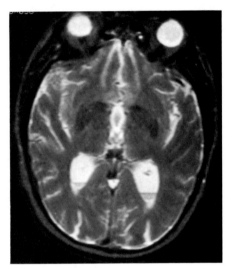

FIG. 66D. SE 2,800/90.

Clinical History

A 67-year-old man with severe headaches.

Findings

The dual-echo pairs of images at the level of the pons and third ventricle (Figs. 66A–D) reveal the presence of fluid-fluid levels within the dependent portion of the occipital horns (Figs. 66A and C, *arrows*). Also note the appearance of rather striking low signal intensity in the superior cerebellar cistern on the second echo image (Fig. 66B). The content of the sediment in the floor of the occipital horns is also relatively low in signal intensity. The T1-weighted coronal images verify the presence of subarachnoid blood, including a focal collection within the superior cerebellar cistern (Figs. 66E and F).

Diagnosis

Recent subarachnoid bleed, with intraventricular reflux.

Discussion

This case was done after the installation of flow compensation gradients into the MR instrument used. The preferential low signal intensity in the superior cerebellar cistern, therefore, is more easily ascribable to the presence of a substance with T2 shortening effect at this field strength (1.5 T) than to pulsation. Of interest, the relative low intensity of the signal here is more striking than that of the sediment in the occipital horns. This may be due to the fact that clot retraction was more easily achieved in this compartment than in the ventricular system given the relatively greater pulsation within. Nevertheless, the red blood cell-containing sediment nicely exhibits the "hematocrit effect" first described in the CT literature for blood within the ventricular system. Its relatively high signal intensity on the first echo images (Figs. 66A and C) is due to the higher protein content of the sediment when compared with normal cerebrospinal fluid.

Ventricular reflux is commonly observed in subarachnoid hemorrhage, particularly when the origin is in the posterior fossa. The blood gains access to the ventricular system through the foramina of Monro and Luschka.

Reference

1. Gomori JN, Grossman RI. Mechanisms responsible for the MR appearance and evolution of intracranial hemorrhage. *Radiographics* 1988;8:427–454.

Submitted by: Michael Brant-Zawadzki, M.D., Senior Editor.

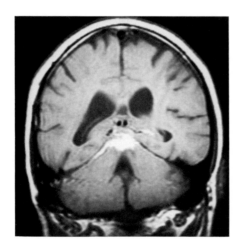

FIG. 66E. SE 800/20.

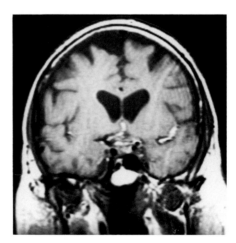

FIG. 66F. SE 800/20.

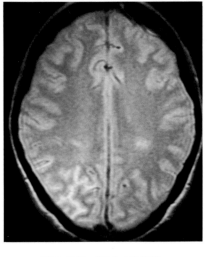

FIG. 67A. SE 2,800/30.

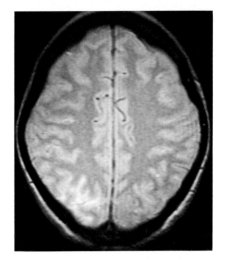

FIG. 67B. SE 2,800/30.

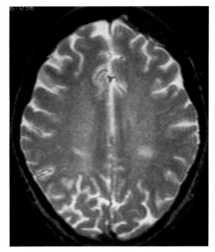

FIG. 67C. 2,800/80.

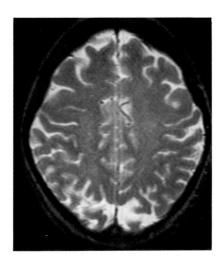

FIG. 67D. SE 2,800/80.

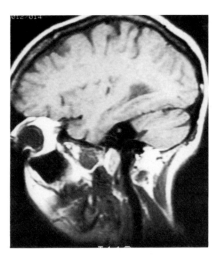

FIG. 67E. SE 600/20.

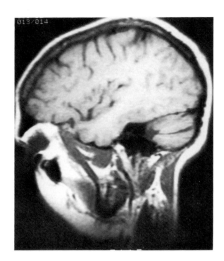

FIG. 67F. SE 600/20.

Clinical History

A 60-year-old woman with acute onset of excruciating headache.

Findings

The first echo images from the long spin-echo sequence (Figs. 67A and B) reveal gyriform areas of elevated signal intensity in the right parietal convexity. Note the difficulty in separating these from normal sulci on the second echo samplings of these same levels (Figs. 66C and D). The T1-weighted sagittal images through this portion of the right hemisphere (Figs. 67E and F) fail to reveal any distinct abnormality. The CT scan obtained the same day shows increased density within the sulci of this right hemispheric region.

Diagnosis

Subarachnoid hemorrhage, verified by lumbar puncture.

Discussion

This case helps illustrate the fact that acute subarachnoid hemorrhage may be very difficult to specifically identify on MR images in the early stage. This is due to the admixture of oxyhemoglobin-containing red blood cells and cerebrospinal fluid (CSF), which may be pulsating. The combination may leave the CSF with relatively low signal intensity indistinguishable from normal CSF, or may only minimally shorten the T1 to such a degree that the normally low intensity of CSF becomes isointense, as in this case. The first echo of the dual-echo sequences may be a clue, but any proteinaceous exudate could produce this. Also, the serpentine structure of the sulci filled with such a fluid may mimic the appearance of edematous gyri.

It is thought that the relatively high oxygen content of the CSF precludes early deoxyhemoglobin formation, which would result in the typical T2 shortening seen with recent hemorrhage. Also, the inability of the liquid CSF-subarachnoid bleed admixture to form a clot precludes the T2-shortening effects of fibrin formation and clot retraction. Thus, CT scanning remains the modality of choice when evaluating patients for acute subarachnoid hemorrhage, a syndrome with relatively specific clinical presentation (acute onset of excruciating headache, stiff neck, and photophobia).

References

1. Bradley WG, Schmidt PG. Effect of methemoglobin formation on the MR appearance of subarachnoid hemorrhage. *Radiology* 1985;156:99–103.
2. Hayman LA, Taber KH, Ford JJ, et al. Effect of clot formation and retraction on spin-echo MR images of blood: an in vitro study. *AJNR* 1989;10:1155–1158.

Submitted by: Michael Brant-Zawadzki, M.D., Senior Editor.

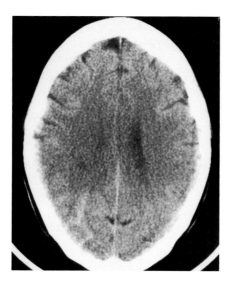

FIG. 67G. CT.

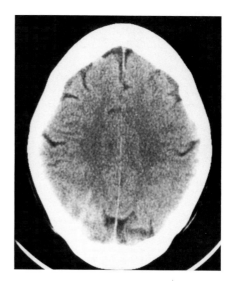

FIG. 67H. CT.

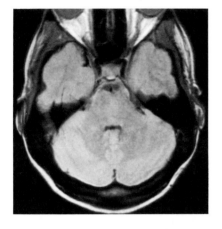

FIG. 68A. SE 2,000/20.

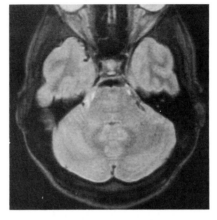

FIG. 68B. SE 2,000/70.

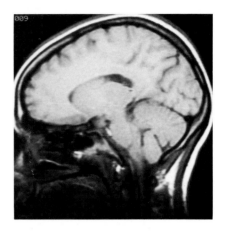

FIG. 68C. SE 600/25.

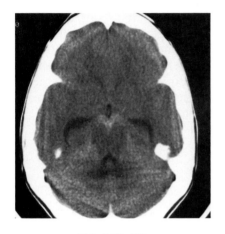

FIG. 68D. CT.

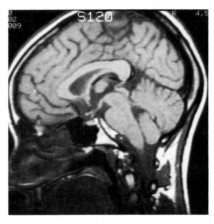

FIG. 68E. SE 600/25.

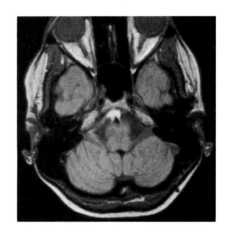

FIG. 68F. SE 2,000/20.

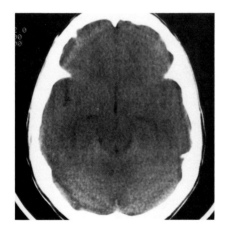

FIG. 68G. CT.

Clinical History

A 26-year-old woman with acute onset of severe headache.

Findings

Magnetic resonance images at the level of the pons obtained with T2-weighted sequences (Figs. 68A and B) reveal a relatively normal appearance, except for obvious low signal intensity surrounding the basilar artery, possibly representing pulsation phenomenon (spin dephasing due to cerebrospinal fluid and basilar artery pulsation). The sagittal T1-weighted image (Fig. 68C) shows a small focus of high signal in the immediate prepontine space. The CT scan (Fig. 68D) leaves little doubt as to the presence of subarachnoid hemorrhage in the interpeduncular cistern. Incidentally noted is the early dilatation of the temporal horns, suggesting early communicating hydrocephalus. On a T2-weighted axial study obtained three weeks later, a high-signal collection is seen immediately anterior to the basilar artery (Fig. 68F), which, on T1-weighted sagittal sequence (Fig. 68E), shows itself as a tubular area of high signal as well. Of interest, the CT scan is relatively unremarkable at this time (Fig. 68G).

Diagnosis

Evolution of subarachnoid hemorrhage from acute to subacute stage.

Discussion

Although it is tempting to ascribe the low signal intensity on the original T2-weighted axial images in the prepontine space (Figs. 68A and B) to the T2 relaxation-shortening effect of deoxyhemoglobin from acute subarachnoid hemorrhage, it is well known that pulsation-induced spin dephasing can produce such low signal intensity, particularly on sequences in which flow compensation gradients are not used (as in this case from 1986). Again, as in the previous case, the point is that fresh subarachnoid hemorrhage can be difficult to identify specifically on MR scanning as compared with CT. However, in the more subacute phase, where blood loses its x-ray attenuating properties (Fig. 68G), the MR scan can be quite helpful by showing the focal clot with its typical shortened T1 relaxation value producing high signal intensity, translating to similar high signal on the second echo image.

Reference

1. Sato HS, Kadoya S. Magnetic resonance imaging of subarachnoid hemorrhage. *Neuroradiology* 1988;30:361–366.

Submitted by: Robert Jahnke, M.D., Lovelace Clinic, Albuquerque, New Mexico; Michael Brant-Zawadzki, M.D., Senior Editor.

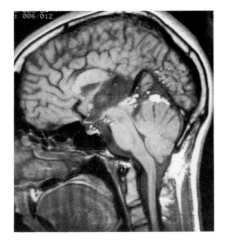

FIG. 69A. SE 800/20.

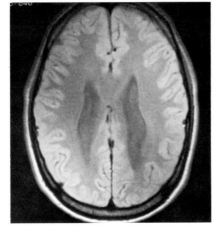

FIG. 69B. SE 2,500/20.

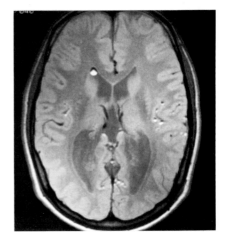

FIG. 69C. SE 2,500/20.

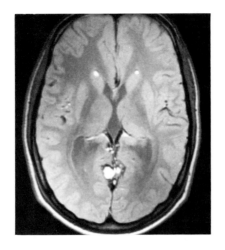

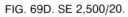

FIG. 69D. SE 2,500/20.

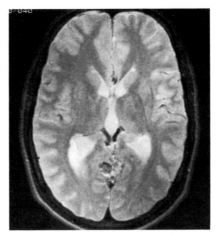

FIG. 69E. SE 2,500/70.

Clinical History

Headache: a 21-year-old man with a history of unspecified low spinal surgery at birth.

Findings

The midsagittal, T1-weighted sequence (Fig. 69A) shows droplets of high signal intensity most prominently distributed through the superior cerebellar cistern, the quadrigeminal plate cistern, the intrapeduncular cistern, and the suprasellar cistern. Associated with this is agenesis of the posterior part of the corpus callosum, with enlargement of a high-riding third ventricle seen. Although the high signal is transiently suggestive of subarachnoid hemorrhage, the dual-echo sequences (Figs. 69B–E) verify the fat-like nature of the droplets in the superior cerebellar cistern, as well as elsewhere in the subarachnoid space and in the right frontal horn of the ventricular system. Also noted is the lack of corpus callosum, the third ventricle rising high to separate the internal cerebral veins. The lateral ventricular bodies are dysplastically large and show separation posteriorly, typical of a corpus callosum agenesis. The chemical shift phenomenon around the high-signal droplets can be seen best on the first echo, the loss of signal intensity between the first and the second echo also typifying fat on these images (Figs. 69D and E).

Incidentally noted is cerebellar ectopia below the foramen magnum, typical for the Chiari I malformation in this patient.

Diagnosis

Partial corpus callosum agenesis, ruptured lipoma superior cerebellar cistern, and Chiari I.

Discussion

Lipomas of the brain's midline are common congenital malformations. These occur in the first 6 to 10 weeks of embryonic life, with inclusion of the mesodermal component during neural tube closure. Other midline disorders, such as corpus callosum agenesis (partial or complete), can accompany their appearance. Ventricular dysplasia, cerebellar ectopia is in the spectrum of these disorders as well. Most often, such abnormalities are found in childhood, but occasionally may go unrecognized until adulthood, as in this case. With fatty lesions in the brain's midline, teratoma comes to mind. Most often, such lesions are in the pineal region and contain calcium as well as cyst and solid components. Teratomas, lipomas, and dermoids can rupture into the subarachnoid space, resulting in the clinical syndrome of chemical meningitis.

Patients with dysplastic lesions in the brain's midline should undergo scanning of the spine as coexistent spinal lesions may exist (hydromyelia, posterior fusion abnormalities, even spinal lipomas or lipomyeloschisis).

The history of neonatal lumbosacral meningocele repair was subsequently obtained, completing the picture of midline dysraphism in this patient with a "forme fruste" of Chiari malformation.

References

1. Barkovich J, et al. Anomalies of the corpus callosum, correlation with further anomalies of the brain. *AJNR* 1988;9:493–501.
2. Barkovich J, et al. Significance of cerebellar tonsillar position on MR. *AJNR* 1986;7:795–799.
3. Kendall B. Dysgenesis of the corpus callosum. *Neuroradiology* 1983;25:239–256.
4. Zettner W, et al. Lipoma of the corpus callosum. *J Neuropathol Exp Neurol* 1960;19:305.

Submitted by: Michael Brant-Zawadzki, M.D., Senior Editor.

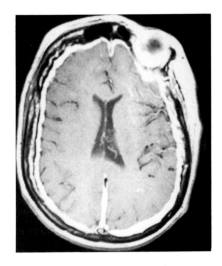

FIG. 70A. SE 800/20.

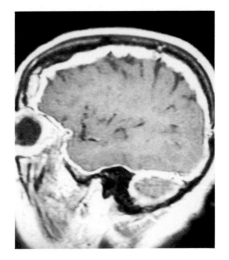

FIG. 70B. SE 600/20.

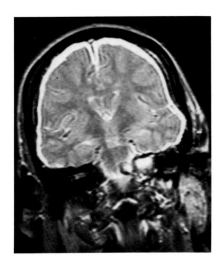

FIG. 70C. SE 2,800/30.

Clinical History

A 71-year-old woman, status postresection of neurinoma 14 years ago, with headaches.

Findings

This study was done following intravenous paramagnetic contrast injection to look for recurrent neurinoma. The incidental finding shown on the T1-weighted axial (Fig. 70A) and sagittal (Fig. 70B) images is the diffuse thickening and homogeneous enhancement of the dura. On the T2-weighted coronal study (Fig. 70C), this simulates a moderate extra-axial fluid collection. Note the regular, relatively smooth edge of the enhancing dura (unlike the case of dural lymphoma in this volume).

Diagnosis

Chronic dural thickening, postoperative.

Discussion

Although the normal dura does not typically show enhancement with paramagnetic contrast, dura that has reacted to a wide variety of insults can do so. This is caused by thickening of the dura with inflammation from prior surgery, bleeding, infection, or intrathecal chemotherapy, or due to the chronic irritation of an indwelling ventricular peritoneal shunt. The dura is a very reactive tissue, with thickening and hyperemia readily occurring due to these insults. Once this occurs, the thickened dura may simulate a chronic subdural fluid collection on MR images without intravenous contrast administration. Following contrast, however, the thickened reactive dura will enhance quite vividly as compared with subdural fluid collections, which should not enhance with contrast (with the exception of subdural empyema, in which the dura also becomes thickened and inflamed).

Additional history in this patient was not just that of craniotomy and ventricular peritoneal shunting following resection of a large acoustic neurinoma (a small remnant of which is seen on the coronal sequence as shown); a history of radiation therapy was also obtained in conjunction with the partial tumor resection. Radiation therapy may aggravate the dural thickening.

References

1. Kilgore D, et al. Cranial tissues: normal MR appearance after intravenous injection of Gd-DTPA. *Radiology* 1986;160:757–761.
2. Berry I, et al. Gd-DTPA in clinical MRI of the brain: II. Extra-axial lesions and normal structures. *AJNR* 1986;7:789–793.
3. Sze G. Personal communication.

Submitted by: Michael Brant-Zawadzki, M.D., Senior Editor.

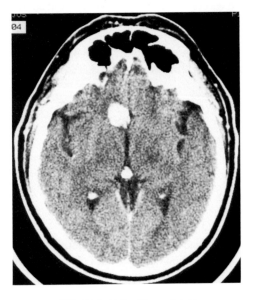

FIG. 71A. CT with contrast.

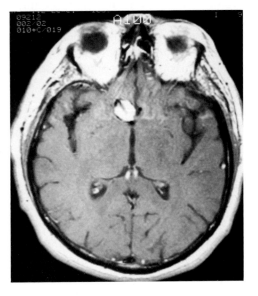

FIG. 71B. SE 800/20 with Gd-DTPA.

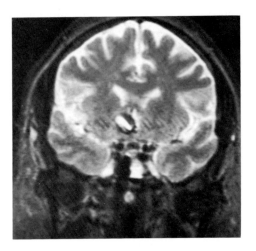

FIG. 71C. SE 2,800/90.

Clinical History

A 63-year-old man with lung carcinoma. A brain scan was ordered for possible metastatic disease screening.

Findings

The original CT study showed an enhancing lesion in the paramedian right subfrontal region (Fig. 71A). The MR scan done with contrast shows a similar lesion in the T1-weighted axial sequence (Fig. 71B). The lesion is also shown on the T2-weighted coronal study (Fig. 71C). Note the tubular low signal intensity entering the lesion on the axial image, and the suggestion of phase dispersion phenomenon from the lesion on both the axial and coronal images. This suggests the possibility of aneurysm with pulsatile flow, which was verified on the gradient-echo flow-sensitive sequence (Fig. 71D) and the angiogram (Fig. 71E).

Diagnosis

Giant aneurysm, resembling metastatic lesion on the contrast-enhanced study.

Discussion

This case illustrates the importance of understanding and identifying flow phenomena on routine MR imaging, as well as the value of flow-sensitive MR sequences in verifying the presence of vascular lesions. Giant aneurysms contain relatively slow flow and may therefore exhibit enhancement with paramagnetic contrast agents similar to that seen in highly vascular solid tumors. Nevertheless, their pulsatile behavior allows phase artifact propagation from their core. Also, sufficient flow through these lesions exists to allow flow-sensitive sequences to detect such flow. In this case, flow-related enhancement within the aneurysm is shown on the gradient-echo sequence (SE 150/15, flip angle 50°, 3 mm slice thickness). Occasionally, thrombus within the lumen of the aneurysm could simulate flow on such a sequence given the high signal intensity from the methemoglobin, which would also appear bright. Therefore, the combination of various phenomena is important to appreciate to definitely detect the presence of flow within such lesions.

References

1. Yousen DM, Balakrishnan J, Debrun GN, et al. Hyperintense thrombus on GRASS MR images: potential pitfall in flow evaluation. *Am J Radiol* 1990;11:51–58.
2. Atlas SW, Goldberg HI, et al. Partially thrombosed giant intracranial aneurysms: correlation of MR and pathologic findings. *Radiology* 1987;162:111–114.

Submitted by: Michael Brant-Zawadzki, M.D., Senior Editor.

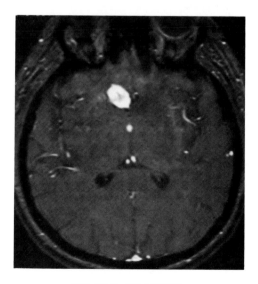

FIG. 71D. SE 150/15.

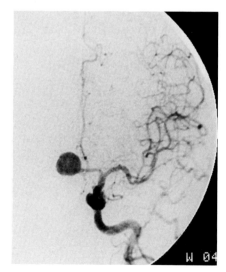

FIG. 71E. Angiogram.

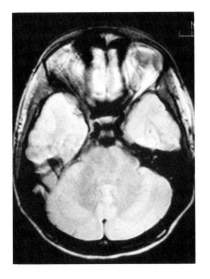

FIG. 72A. SE 2,500/30.

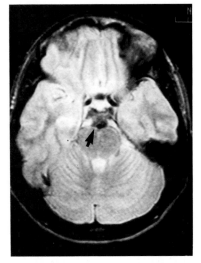

FIG. 72B. SE 2,500/30.

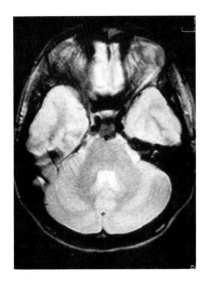

FIG. 72C. SE 2,500/60.

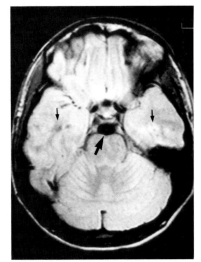

FIG. 72D. SE 2,500/60.

Clinical History

A 30-year-old man with severe headache.

Findings

Axial T2-W (SE 2,500/30 and 60) images are provided. The first echo images show a rounded, low-signal region in the pontine cistern in the region of the tip of basilar artery (Fig. 72B, *arrow*). The second echo images show that the low signal region now fills in with intermediate signal (Fig. 72D, *arrow*). The signal-void basilar artery is now well seen interfaced with the intermediate signal in the prepontine cistern.

High-signal amorphous regions are seen in the left temporal lobe, and low-signal regions are seen in the right (Fig. 72A). These temporal-lobe signal abnormalities are directly lateral to the low-signal region in the pontine cistern.

Diagnosis

Basilar artery pseudoaneurysm secondary to motion artifact.

Discussion

Cerebrospinal fluid (CSF) motion from transmitted vascular pulsations can result in focal areas of CSF hypointensity on MR images because of signal mismapping from phase shift. When this CSF flow void occurs adjacent to the basilar artery in the pontine cistern, it may be mistaken for a basilar artery aneurysm on proton-density and T2-weighted images. The flow artifact is most common in the pediatric population, in which younger, more pliable vessels transmit pulsations more easily than do less elastic, atherosclerotic vessels of older individuals.

Reference

1. Burt TB. MR of CSF flow mimicking basilar artery aneurysm. *AJNR* 1987;8:55–58.

Submitted by: Louis M. Teresi, M.D., Stephen J. Davis, M.D., and Mark Ziemba, M.D., Huntington Medical Research Institutes, Pasadena, California; William G. Bradley, Jr., M.D., Ph.D., Senior Editor.

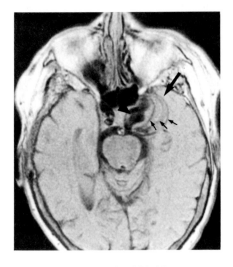

FIG. 73A. SE 800/30.

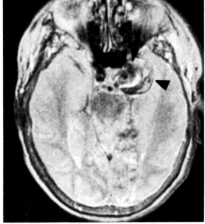

FIG. 73B. SE 2,000/30.

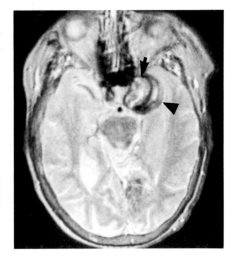

FIG. 73C. SE 3,000/85.

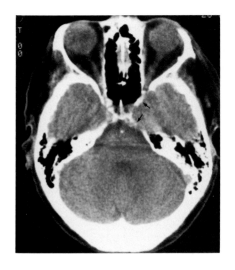

FIG. 73D. CT without contrast.

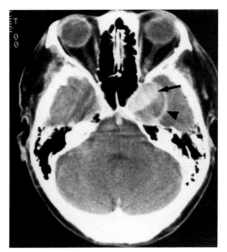

FIG. 73E. CT with contrast.

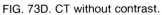

Clinical History

An 82-year-old woman with a history of diplopia.

Findings

Axial T2-W (SE 2,000/30 and SE 3,000/85) and axial T1-W (SE 800/30) images are provided for review. The T1-weighted image shows a large isointense mass apparently arising from the left cavernous sinus (Fig. 73A, *arrow*). The mass has a laminated appearance, with alternating low and isointense bands (Fig. 73A, *small arrows*). The left supraclinoid internal carotid artery appears dilated (Fig. 73A, *arrowhead*). The SE 2,000/30 sequence (Fig. 73B) shows that the periphery (*arrowhead*) of the mass remains nearly isointense to brain; however, the interior (*arrow*) has mixed high- and low-signal areas. The more T2-W SE 3,000/85 sequence (Fig. 73C) shows that the interior (*arrow*) of the mass becomes more intense, whereas the periphery (*arrowhead*) becomes more hypointense.

Non-enhanced CT scan shows mass effect in the left cavernous sinus with remodeling and erosion of the left lateral wall of the sphenoid sinus and petrous apex (Fig. 73D, *arrow*). The contrast-enhanced CT scan shows that the medial aspect of the mass enhances (Fig. 73E, *arrow*), as does its periphery (Fig. 73E, *arrowhead*).

Scattered foci of increased signal intensity are seen in the deep white matter on the right.

Diagnosis

Partially thrombosed aneurysm of the cavernous internal carotid artery.

Discussion

Intracavernous carotid aneurysms constitute approximately 5–8% of all intracranial aneurysms. They are commonly unilateral, but bilateral intracavernous aneurysms are not rare. They may rupture within the cavernous sinus, with formation of an arteriovenous fistula, or in the sphenoid sinus, producing epistaxis. These aneurysms may develop like a slowly expanding, pulsatile parasellar tumor and manifest themselves as a cavernous sinus syndrome, with facial numbness or pain and paresis of extraocular muscles due to pressure effects on the 3rd, 4th, and 6th cranial nerves in the cavernous sinus.

Giant partially thrombosed aneurysms may be more clearly and definitively diagnosed and characterized by MRI than by CT. With CT, a partially enhancing mass with mixed attenuation in non-enhancing regions is usually evident. The enhancement is generally of two varieties: a central round to oval region of homogeneous enhancement extending to one of the margins, which is usually adjacent to a major cerebral artery, and a peripheral-enhancing rim. Calcification may also be evident peripherally. The central enhancement represents the residual lumen. The peripheral enhancement is probably related to organization of the mural thrombus.

Magnetic resonance imaging will usually more clearly reveal the relationship of the residual aneurysm lumen to the parent cerebral artery. This may be seen on spin-echo images as flow voids in the parent vessel and aneurysm or on single-slice gradient-echo images (e.g., GRASS) as high-intensity structures. On spin-echo images, the luminal clot appears as layered areas of mixed, mostly low signal intensity in the chronic phase, as hyperintense signal on both T1- and T2-weighted images in the subacute phase, and as isointense signal on T-1 weighted images and as markedly hypointense signal on T2-weighted images in the acute phase. A variable rim of hyperintense subacute clot is usually apparent on T1-weighted images at the margin of the residual aneurysm lumen and the surrounding thrombosed portion of the lumen. The organized luminal clot is heterogeneously low intensity due to fibrous collagen deposition and the presence of hemosiderin-laden macrophages.

References

1. Olsen WL, Brant-Zawadzki M, Hodes J, et al. Giant intracranial aneurysms: MR imaging. *Radiology* 1987;163:431.
2. Atlas SW, Grossman RI, Goldberg HI, et al. Partially thrombosed giant intracranial aneurysms: correlation of MRI and pathological findings. *Radiology* 1987;162:111–114.

Submitted by: Louis M. Teresi, M.D., Stephen J. Davis, M.D., and Mark Ziemba, M.D., Huntington Medical Research Institutes, Pasadena, California; William G. Bradley, Jr., M.D., Ph.D., Senior Editor.

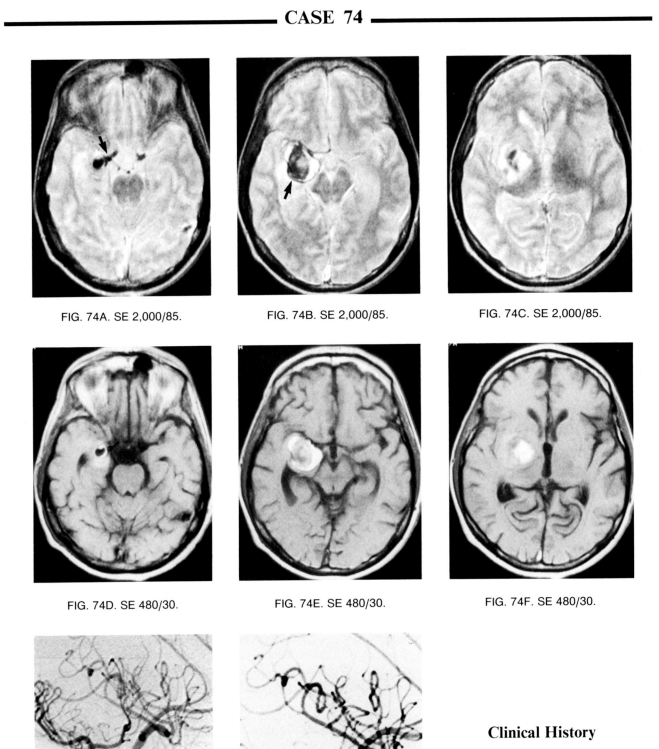

FIG. 74A. SE 2,000/85.

FIG. 74B. SE 2,000/85.

FIG. 74C. SE 2,000/85.

FIG. 74D. SE 480/30.

FIG. 74E. SE 480/30.

FIG. 74F. SE 480/30.

FIG. 74G. Angiogram.

FIG. 74H. Angiogram.

Clinical History

A 43-year-old man with diplopia.

Findings

Axial T2-W (SE 2,000/85) images show an approximately 3 cm mass with a predominantly low-signal center and high-signal peripheral rim medial and inferior to the right temporal lobe (Fig. 74B, *arrow*). The mass displaces the temporal lobe, extends into the right anterolateral thalamus, and deforms the right occipital horn. A low-signal linear structure extends from the mass inferiorly (Fig. 74A, *arrow*). On the T1-weighted images, the periphery of the mass remains high signal; however, the center becomes lower in signal intensity (Figs. 74D–F). The digital arteriogram shows opacification of the lumen of a large posterior communicating artery aneurysm (Fig. 74G, *arrow*). The aneurysm was then occluded with a balloon solidified after positioning with a hema-containing polymer. Digital arteriogram after placement of the balloon shows a thin rim of contrast outlining the balloon in the aneurysm lumen (Fig. 74H, *arrow*).

Diagnosis

Posterior communicating artery aneurysm, post-balloon occlusion.

Discussion

Posterior communicating artery aneurysms comprise 20% of all cerebral berry aneurysms and may present with diplopia from compression of the 3rd cranial nerve in the ambient cistern.

When intracranial aneurysms cannot be clipped, occlusion of the parent artery in an effort to induce aneurysm thrombosis is often appropriate. The use of detachable balloons offers advantages over traditional surgical techniques for inducing aneurysm thrombosis and reducing the risk of hemorrhage. In the postembolization evaluation of intracranial aneurysms, MRI can provide information on the evolution of aneurysmal intraluminal thrombosis, integrity of the embolized aneurysm lumen, associated mass effect, and complications of intravascular therapy (1).

Thrombi occurring in aneurysms as the result of balloon occlusion are initiated primarily by stasis and, consequently, are likely to be more closely related in composition to venous (red) thrombi than to arterial (white) thrombi. Thrombi in patients examined within 48 hours after balloon occlusion have signal intensities consistent with those of nonflowing blood. In the period 5 to 10 days after treatment, as erythrocyte lysis, hemoglobin breakdown, and thrombus organization occur, thrombi assume some of the MR characteristics of parenchymal hematomas. By four to six weeks after treatment, the predominant signal intensity corresponds to that expected for extracellular methemoglobin. In general, tissue with a signal corresponding to that of hemosiderin is less prominent than in parenchymal hematomas of corresponding volume.

To date, there is limited experience in the MR appearance of the balloon itself. Most polymers for endovascular therapy have intermediate T1 and T2 values. Hema-containing polymers, as the one used in this case, may show T2 shortening because of the heme elements in the polymer.

References

1. Strother CM, Eldevik P, Kikuchi Y, et al. Thrombous formation and structure and evolution of mass effect in intracranial aneurysms treated by balloon embolization: emphasis on MR findings. *AJNR* 1989;10:787–796.
2. Fox AJ, Vinuela F, Pelz DM, et al. Use of detachable balloons for proximal artery occlusion in the treatment of unclippable cerebral aneurysms. *J Neurosurg* 1987;66:40–46.
3. Atlas SW, Grossman RI, Goldberg HI, et al. Partially thrombosed giant intracranial aneurysms: correlation of MRI and pathological findings. *Radiology* 1987;162:111–114.

Submitted by: Louis M. Teresi, M.D., Stephen J. Davis, M.D., and Mark Ziemba, M.D., Huntington Medical Research Institutes, Pasadena, California; William G. Bradley, Jr., M.D., Ph.D., Senior Editor.

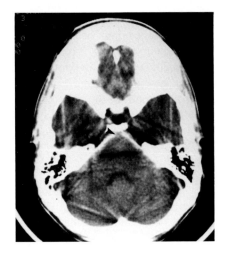

FIG. 75A. CT.

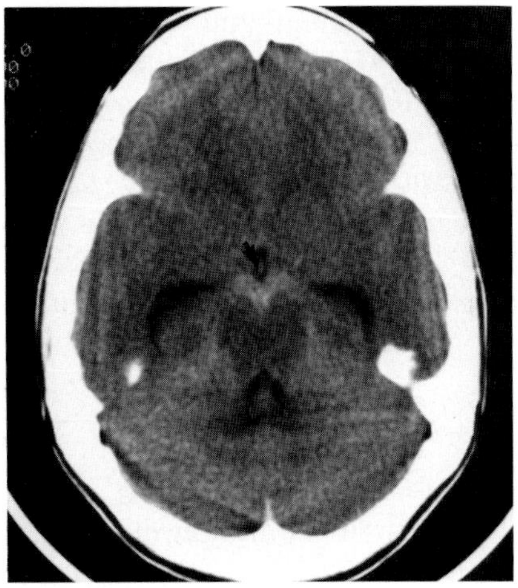

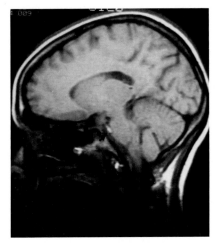

FIG. 75C. SE 600/25.

FIG. 75B. CT.

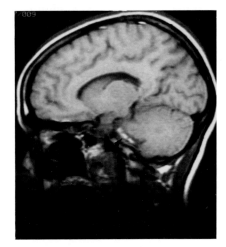

FIG. 75D. SE 600/25.

176

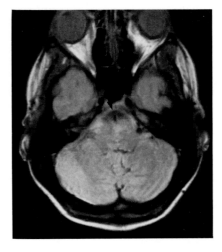

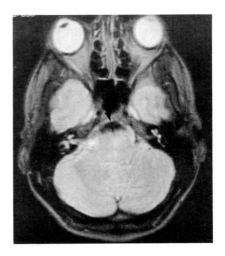

FIG. 75E. SE 2,000/20.

FIG. 75F. SE 2,000/70.

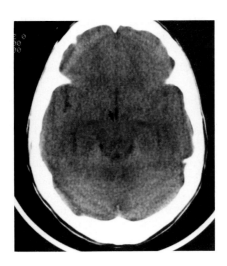

FIG. 75G. CT.

Clinical History

A 26-year-old woman with severe headache and stiff neck.

Axial T2-W (SE 2,000/20 and 70) and sagittal T1-W (SE 600/25) images from both July 7 and July 29 are provided for review. A non-contrast CT scan from July 4 is also provided and shows a marked beam-hardening artifact in the pontine cistern (Fig. 75A); however, dense material in the interpeduncular cistern, consistent with subarachnoid hemorrhage, is noted (Fig. 75B, *arrow*). Sagittal SE 600/25 MR images from July 7 show hyperintense material in the pontine and ambient cisterns (Figs. 75C and D, *arrows*). Axial SE 2,000/20 and SE 2,000/70 images show decreased signal intensity in the pontine cistern, more hypointense on the SE 2,000/70 images (Figs. 75E and F, *arrows*). The repeat non-contrast CT from July 8 shows that the high-density material in the interpeduncular cistern is now intermediate density (Fig. 75G, *arrow*). The sagittal SE 600/25 images from July 29 show increased signal in the pontine cistern (Fig. 75H, *arrows*). The axial SE 2,000/20 and SE 2,000/70 images now show high-signal material in the pontine cisterns (Figs. 75I and J, *arrows*).

Diagnosis

Evolution of subarachnoid thrombus.

Discussion

Unlike CT, where detection of subarachnoid hemorrhage in the initial three to five days is apparent and diagnostic in nearly 80–90% of cases, the opposite is true of MR. On CT, the detection of extravasated blood is due to the presence in cerebrospinal fluid (CSF) of the high protein concentration of the globin molecule in the red blood cells. As the blood products are absorbed during the next three to five days, the CT attenuation values also decrease.

On MR, the detection of subarachnoid hemorrhage is also based on the structure of hemoglobin and its various breakdown products as well as on the protein in the plasma. The MR appearance of subarachnoid hemorrhage differs significantly from intraparenchymal, subdural, or epidural hemorrhage due to admixture with CSF. Immediately after subarachnoid hemorrhage, there is a small decrease in T1, which most likely reflects the increase in hydration-layer water due to the elevated protein content of the bloody CSF. As shown in vitro, significant quantities of methemoglobin are not formed until several days after the hemorrhage. Several days to a week post-ictus, signal intensity increases in the subarachnoid space due to methemoglobin formation. In cases of milder subarachnoid hemorrhage, red blood cells may have been resorbed by the time significant methemoglobin formation has occurred, and, therefore, the anticipated short T1 appearance will not be seen. For these reasons, CT is advocated for the early diagnosis of subarachnoid hemorrhage in the clinical setting. The short T2 properties of a hematoma require both the formation of deoxyhemoglobin and clot retraction. For both reasons, the short T2 appearance is rarely observed in subarachnoid hemorrhage unless massive bleeding has occurred, in which case a subarachnoid thrombus is

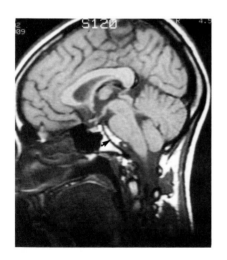

FIG. 75H. SE 600/25.

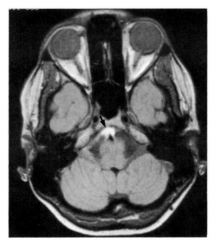

FIG. 75I. SE 2,000/20.

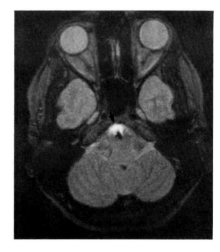

FIG. 75J. SE 2,000/70.

present. In addition, the oxygen tension in the subarachnoid space is higher than that in the center of a hematoma or a tumor; thus, deoxyhemoglobin (and eventually methemoglobin) forms more slowly than in the lower oxygen environments.

Reference

1. Bradley WG, Schmidt PC. Effect of methemoglobin formation of the MR appearance of subarachnoid hemorrhage. *Radiology* 1986;156:99–103.

Submitted by: Louis M. Teresi, M.D. and Stephen J. Davis, M.D., Huntington Medical Research Institutes, Pasadena, California; William G. Bradley, Jr., M.D., Ph.D., Senior Editor.

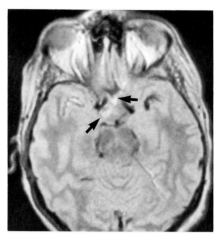

FIG. 76A. SE 3,000/30.

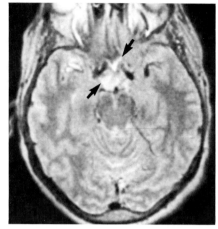

FIG. 76B. SE 3,000/80.

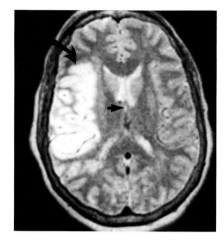

FIG. 76C. SE 3,000/80.

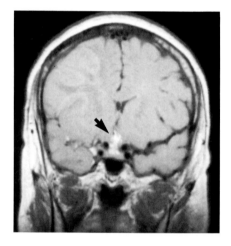

FIG. 76D. SE 750/40.

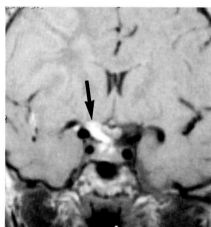

FIG. 76E. SE 750/40.

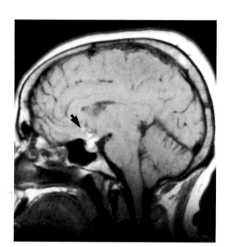

FIG. 76F. SE 500/40.

Clinical History

A 37-year-old woman with acute onset of severe headache, followed by left arm numbness and weakness.

Findings

Axial T2-W (SE 3,000/30 and 80), sagittal T1-W (SE 500/40), and coronal T1-W (SE 750/40) images are provided for review. On the axial T2-weighted images, high signal is noted in the right temporal lobe, extending across white and gray matter (Fig. 76C, *curved arrow*). Mass effect shifts the midline to the left (Fig. 76C, *small arrow*). Subtle increased signal is also seen in the suprasellar cistern on both the SE 3,000/30 (Fig. 76A, *arrows*) and the SE 3,000/80 (Fig. 76B, *arrows*) sequences. The signal intensity is greater than cerebrospinal fluid on both sequences. On the sagittal and coronal T1-weighted sequences (Figs. 76D–F, *arrows*), very high signal material is seen in the suprasellar cistern extending into the sella.

Diagnosis

Subarachnoid hemorrhage with infarction in the right middle cerebral artery distribution.

Discussion

The incidence of positive angiograms in the evaluation of subarachnoid hemorrhage (SAH) varies between 70% and 90%. Aneurysms account for 80% of SAHs and arteriovenous malformations account for 5% (2). The location of subarachnoid clot in this patient in the region of the circle of Willis suggests an aneurysm as a likely cause of the SAH.

The irritative effects of subarachnoid blood on vessels causes spasm, which accounts for the severe headache associated with SAH as well as its most severe complication, cerebral infarction, reported in approximately 35–40% of patients with significant SAH. Vasospasm usually occurs between days 5 and 16 following SAH; however, onset may occur as early as day 3. Although the pathogenesis of vasospasm is unclear, many investigators have noted a correlation between the amount of blood seen on CT and MR and the subsequent development of vasospasm.

References

1. Bradley WG, Schmidt PC. Effect of methemoglobin formation on the MR appearance of subarachnoid hemorrhage. *Radiology* 1985;156:99–103.
2. Bjorkensten G, Halonen V. Incidence of intracranial vascular lesions in patients with subarachnoid hemorrhage investigated by four-vessel angiography. *J Neurosurg* 1965;23:29.

Submitted by: Louis M. Teresi, M.D., Stephen J. Davis, M.D., and Mark Ziemba, M.D., Huntington Medical Research Institutes, Pasadena, California; William G. Bradley, Jr., M.D., Ph.D., Senior Editor.

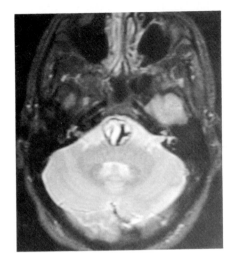

FIG. 77A. SE 2,800/70.

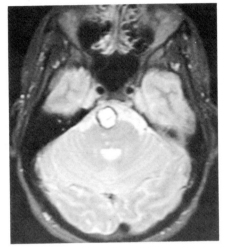

FIG. 77B. SE 2,800/70.

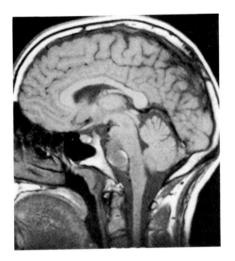

FIG. 77C. SE 500/20.

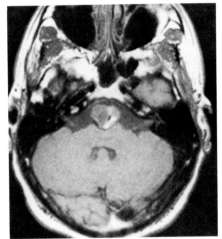

FIG. 77D. SE 600/20.

Clinical History

A 34-year-old man with dizziness.

Findings

T2-weighted axial images (Figs. 77A and B) show a well-circumscribed, 1 cm mass anterior to the pons. Note the low-signal periphery, the high-signal center, and the unusual internal low-signal linear structures. The T1-weighted sagittal and axial images (Figs. 77C and D) show the lesion to be extra-axial, with some curvilinear high-signal components in the periphery and a punctate low-signal intensity in the center noted on the axial image. None of the images depict a normal basilar artery.

Diagnosis

Fusiform aneurysm, basilar artery.

Discussion

The presence of a well-circumscribed lesion in the general distribution of the basilar artery should prompt consideration of an aneurysm. The lack of flow void in the structure does not dissuade one from that diagnosis, as fusiform aneurysms of the basilar artery can thrombose, leaving only a small, if any, remnant lumen for the basilar artery. The peripheral low-signal rim may represent calcification and/or hemosiderin deposition. The central low signal intensity foci may represent channels, fresh clot, or hemosiderin. The admixtures of signal within the structure can make the specific diagnosis difficult. The diagnosis is generally made by exclusion. Epidermoids in this location would tend to have much lower signal intensity on the T1-weighted sequences and not reveal the inhomogeneous signal variations or the peripheral low signal intensity ring. Meningiomas would be much more homogeneous, show a dural base, and reveal more of an isointense signal on the sequences, particularly the second echoes. Other extra-axial lesions would be rare and, in any case, would displace the basilar artery, which might be seen off midline. Occasionally, dolichoectasia of the basilar artery can simulate an aneurysm; however, this arterial enlargement is generally more uniform in nature. Nevertheless, the transmitted pulsations from this ectatic vessel can simulate a larger structure.

The signal intensities within an aneurysmal lumen reflect the combination of blood by-products, whether they be deoxyhemoglobin, methemoglobin, or hemosiderin, as well as flow effects. Signal void due to high-velocity flow or to turbulent dephasing of nuclear spins can occur. Flow-related enhancement can occur under appropriate conditions as well. Therefore, assigning any particular locus of signal intensity to a single pathophysiologic event becomes quite difficult.

References

1. Atlas SW, Grossman RI, Goldberg HI, et al. Partially thrombosed giant intracranial aneurysms: correlation of MR and pathologic findings. *Radiology* 1987;162:111–114.
2. Olsen WL, Brant-Zawadzki M, Hodes J, et al. Giant intracranial aneurysms: MR imaging. *Radiology* 1987;163:431–435.

Submitted by: Walter Kucharczyk, M.D., Toronto General Hospital, Toronto, Canada; Michael Brant-Zawadzki, M.D., Senior Editor.

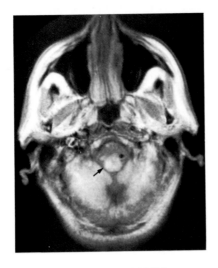

FIG. 78A. SE 2,200/30.

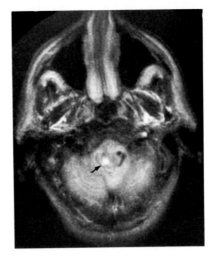

FIG. 78B. SE 2,200/100.

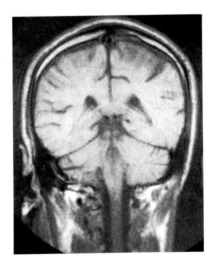

FIG. 78C. SE 683/26.

Clinical History

A 56-year-old man with acute onset of left leg weakness.

Findings

Axial T2-W (SE 2,200/30 and 100) and coronal T1-W (SE 683/26) images are provided for review. The T2-weighted axial images show a focus of increased signal intensity (*arrows*) in the lower right medulla on both the first (Fig. 78A) and second (Fig. 78B) echo studies. The lesion is not seen on the T1-weighted coronal study (Fig. 78C).

Diagnosis

Brainstem infarction involving the corticospinal tract.

Discussion

Motor function to the body and face is carried in the corticospinal and corticobulbar tracts, which start in the precentral (motor) cortex. The axons of the corticospinal tracts are the longest in the body, extending from the motor cortex as far caudad as the lower thoracic cord. All motor fibers descend through the corona radiata and the internal capsule. These fibers subsequently pass through the cerebral pedicles of the midbrain, where some of the corticobulbar fibers cross to supply the contralateral motor nuclei of cranial nerves III and IV, supplying all the extraocular muscles except the lateral rectus. Motor fibers continue to descend through the tegmentum of the pons, the corticobulbar fibers crossing at the level of the 4th ventricle to supply the motor nuclei of the 3rd division of the trigeminal nerve (CN V) as well as the abducens nucleus (CN VI) and the facial nerve nuclei (CN VII). In the medulla, fibers from the corticobulbar tracts cross to supply the motor nuclei of cranial nerves IX through XII.

In the basilar portion of the pons, the corticospinal tracts become confluent and are generally visible on MR images as rounded structures on the ventral aspect of the brainstem.

At the cervicomedullary junction, most of the corticospinal fibers cross as they descend into the spinal cord. Because of this decussation, lesions of the corticospinal tract above the decussation lead to contralateral hemiparesis in the body, whereas those below lead to ipsilateral hemiparesis. The lesion in this case is located above the level of the decussation and, therefore, causes a contralateral hemiparesis.

References

1. Flannigan BD, Bradley WG, et al. Magnetic resonance imaging of the brainstem: normal structure and basic functional anatomy. *Radiology* 1985;154:375–384.
2. Bradley WG. MRI of the brainstem: state of the art. *Radiology.* (In press.)
3. Clark RG. *Manter and Gatz's essentials of neuroanatomy and neurophysiology.* Philadelphia: FA Davis, 1979.

Submitted by: Louis M. Teresi, M.D., Stephen J. Davis, M.D., and Mark Ziemba, M.D., Huntington Medical Research Institutes, Pasadena, California; William G. Bradley, Jr., M.D., Ph.D., Senior Editor.

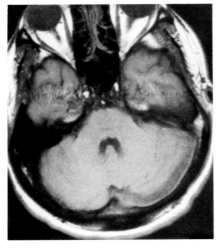

FIG. 79A. SE 700/20.

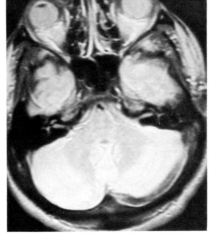

FIG. 79B. SE 2,800/35.

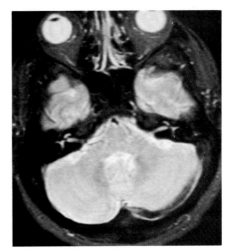

FIG. 79C. SE 2,800/70.

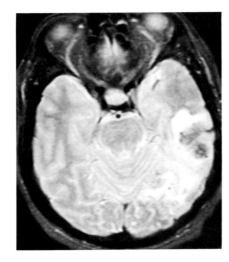

FIG. 79D. SE 2,800/70.

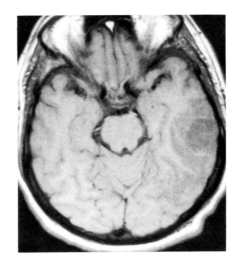

FIG. 79E. SE 700/20.

Clinical History

Sudden altered state of consciousness, aphasia, and right-sided weakness in a 28-year-old man.

Findings

Axial sequences at the level of the left transverse sinus show low signal intensity within that structure on all three images obtained with T1 weighting as well as both echoes obtained using the T2-weighted technique (Figs. 79A–C). In addition, the higher sections demonstrate a mass lesion in the left temporal lobe that shows mixed signal characteristics. The T1-weighted sequence shows low signal intensity in the periphery of the left temporal lobe, surrounded by a serpentine-appearing distorted low signal intensity structure of the underlying brain. The second echo at the same level of the T2-weighted sequence shows preferential low signal intensity within the peripheral mass component and high signal intensity in the subjacent white matter (Figs. 79D and E).

Diagnosis

Acute transverse sinus thrombosis, with resulting venous infarct of the left temporal lobe.

Discussion

This case emphasizes the difficulty in making the diagnosis of dural sinus thrombosis in an acute phase. The signal intensity one might expect (that is, high signal) from a clot in the dural sinus is absent here. The low signal intensity is explainable on the basis of magnetic susceptibility effects of fresh clot, emphasized by the high field strength (1.5 T). Also, clot retraction and fibrin accumulation can lead to such T2 shortening as well as lower field strengths. Isolated transverse sinus thrombosis can occur, particularly when in the setting of mastoid infection (not present in this case). Resulting venous thrombosis occurs due to propagation of clot into the cortical veins, which drain into the transverse sinus such as the vein of Labbe, a major draining vein for the temporal lobe. The resulting cessation of drainage produces increased pressure in the capillary system, which predisposes to rupture. The combined etiologies of decreased perfusion (no outflow) and hemorrhage will produce the hemorrhage infarct shown here.

References

1. Hayman LA, Taber KH, Ford JJ, et al. Effective clot formation and retraction on spin-echo MR images of blood: an in vitro study. *AJNR* 1989;10:1155–1158.
2. Hecht-Leavitt C, Gomori JN, Grossman RI. High field MRI of hemorrhagic cortical infarction. *AJNR* 1986;7:581–585.
3. McArdle CB, Mirfakhraee MM, Amparo EG. MR imaging of transverse/sigmoid dural sinus and jugular vein thrombosis. *J Comput Assist Tomogr* 1987;11:831–838.

Submitted by: Walter Kucharczyk, M.D., Toronto General Hospital, Toronto, Canada; Michael Brant-Zawadzki, M.D., Senior Editor.

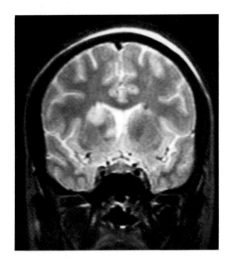

FIG. 80A. September 10, 1988, SE 2,800/80.

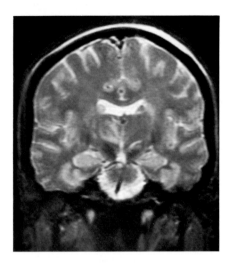

FIG. 80B. September 10, 1988, SE 2,800/80.

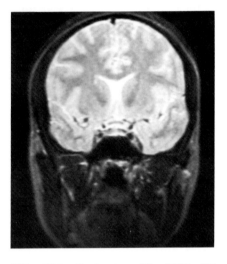

FIG. 80C. September 16, 1988, SE 2,800/70.

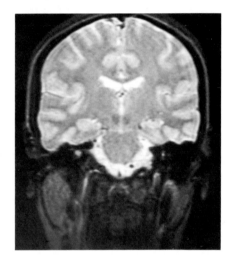

FIG. 80D. September 16, 1988, SE 2,800/70.

Clinical History

A 24-year-old woman, one day postpartum, with seizure, impaired upward gaze, and mild leg weakness. Her pregnancy was complicated by pre-eclampsia, which was treated with magnesium sulfate.

Findings

The MRI scan obtained one day after admission shows abnormalities in the pons, right thalamus, and region of the caudate nucleus and internal capsule consisting of high-signal alteration of the normal structures. At this point, multifocal infarction was considered on the basis of hypercoagulable state resulting from the recent pregnancy. However, the neurologic symptoms resolved and the patient was re-scanned six days later. Note the complete clearing of the lesions from the affected sites on the T2-weighted images (Figs. 80C and D).

Diagnosis

Transient "edema" of eclampsia.

Discussion

A number of recent case reports have documented the finding of reversible brain abnormalities in young women with eclampsia. The clinical presentation of this patient is quite typical. The predominant theory for central nervous system dysfunction is based on the occurrence of a combination of vasculopathy with vessel wall damage, intracerebral hemorrhage, hypoxic-ischemic brain damage, and cerebral edema. Although large hemorrhages may occur, multiple small intracerebral hemorrhages are more common. Hypoxic-ischemic changes, as evidenced by the histologic features of the ischemic cell process, are predominantly limited to the cortex, but they may involve gray–white matter junctional regions.

In several of the reported cases, however, the overall picture was much more benign, with the initially abnormal brain changes resolving to a more normal appearance. Whether this represents transient "breakthrough" edema due to vascular bed disruption produced by the hypertensive process or transient ischemic edema secondary to spasm/vasculopathy in these cases is not understood.

References

1. Schwaighofer B, et al. MR demonstration of reversible brain abnormalities in eclampsia. *J Comput Assist Tomogr* 1989;13:310–312.
2. Fredriksson S, et al. Repeated cranial computed tomographic and magnetic resonance imaging scans in two cases of eclampsia. *Stroke* 1989;20:547–553.
3. Dierckx I. MR findings in eclampsia. *AJNR* 1989;10:445.

Submitted by: Michael Brant-Zawadzki, M.D., Senior Editor.

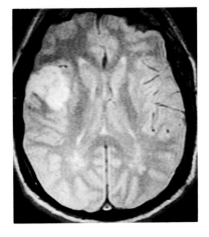

FIG. 81A. January 13, 1989; SE 2,800/30.

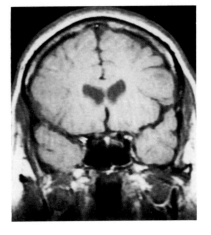

FIG. 81B. January 13, 1989; SE 800/20.

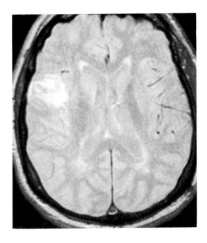

FIG. 81C. April 18, 1989; SE 2,800/30.

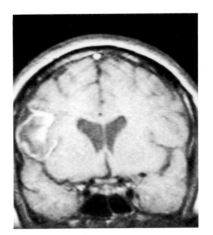

FIG. 81D. April 18, 1989; SE 600/30.

Clinical History

A 60-year-old man. Initial study (January 13, 1989) was done for left-sided weakness; the subsequent study (April 18, 1989) was done for right arm numbness and tingling.

Findings

The T2-weighted axial, first echo image (Fig. 81A) of the initial study shows a focal area of elevated signal intensity within the anterior middle cerebral artery distribution. Note the relative sparing of the white matter, the signal intensity predominating in the gray matter structures. There is a mass effect that is shown well by the coronal T1-weighted image (Fig. 81B).

The subsequent study done in April documents that the lesion decreased in overall volume. There is a serpentine elevation of signal intensity in the periphery of the lesion as well as in its medial border. Note the interval decrease in overall mass effect and the slight enlargement of the right lateral ventricle.

Diagnosis

Evolution of acute ischemic infarct, with secondary petechial hemorrhage developing over time.

Discussion

The initial study shows the typical appearance of a right middle cerebral artery branch infarction. The predominant involvement of the gray matter is a strong clue to the nature of the lesion. A tumor could have this appearance, but would be expected to involve the white matter as well. The good geographic distribution for anterior opercular branches of the middle cerebral artery fits with the impression of a vascular event. The mass effect indicates the early phase of infarction (days 2–5). The subsequent study done for a new symptom shows what at first might appear to be a worrisome event—that of hemorrhagic transformation of the right middle cerebral artery infarction. However, this is a typical pathophysiologic evolutionary event. As blood flow is re-established to the infarcted brain, and before normal autoregulatory mechanisms can be reestablished in the damaged brain tissue, normal systemic pressure is introduced into the damaged vascular bed and small amounts of petechial hemorrhage may occur. This typically is seen in small branch infarcts, such as this one, in the second or third week following the event. Such petechial hemorrhages may persist for months (as in this case). Their appearance is not a contraindication to continued anticoagulation or an indication of reinfarction. In fact, these small bleeds are typically silent clinically, discovered only incidentally when MR imaging is performed. The incidence of such secondary petechial hemorrhage on a delayed basis into infarction is as high as 42%. The high signal intensity results from the methemoglobin component of the hemorrhage.

It should be noted that large, proximal embolic occlusions of the middle cerebral artery, which result in major infarction, are predisposed to more acute hemorrhage in the first few days following the infarct, particularly if anticoagulation is used. Such hemorrhagic complications in the acute phase of infarction can produce a clinical deterioration of the patient.

References

1. Okata AY, Yamaguchi T, Mineamtsu K, et al. *Stroke* 1989;20:598–603.
2. Horning CR, Dorndorf W, Agnolia L. Hemorrhagic infarction—a prospective study. *Stroke* 1986;17:179–185.

Submitted by: Michael Brant-Zawadzki, M.D., Senior Editor.

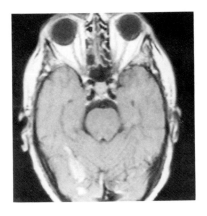
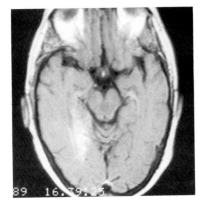
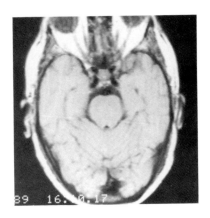

FIG. 82A. SE 805/32 with Gd-DTPA.   FIG. 82B. SE 805/32 with Gd-DTPA.   FIG. 82C. SE 805/32.

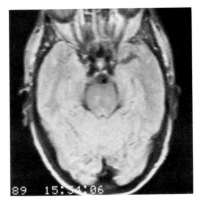
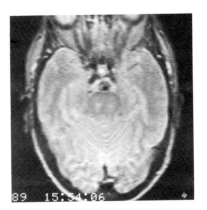

FIG. 82D. SE 2,500/48.   FIG. 82E. SE 2,500/96.

Clinical History

Sudden onset of visual disturbance and headache, with no focal neurologic signs. Scan was obtained four days later.

Findings

The T1-weighted images obtained after intravenous administration of gadolinium-DTPA (Figs. 82A and B) reveal enhancement in the general distribution of the posterior temporal artery, including the posterior hippocampus and undersurface of the occipital lobe in the right hemisphere. Note the absence of mass effect. The pre-contrast T1-weighted image fails to reveal any abnormality (Fig. 82C). This is also true of the dual-echo T2-weighted axial images (Figs. 82D and E). No obvious elevation of signal intensity is seen, and no edema is noted in the area of enhancement shown in Figs. 82A and B.

Diagnosis

Subacute infarct, seen only with contrast enhancement.

Discussion

Contrast enhancement in infarction certainly occurs, particularly after the first 48 hours, when blood-brain barrier disruption has occurred and reperfusion is established to the area of infarction. In all such instances, some degree of edema will accompany the pathophysiologic process resulting in high signal intensity on the T2-weighted images. However, in occasional instances, there is insufficient hydrostatic pressure within the area of infarction to produce significant brain edema, or, possibly, white blood cell infiltration of the infarct shortens the T1 relaxation of the edema that does develop. Also possible is the leakage of sufficient serum protein in the area of infarction along with the edema, to counterbalance the prolongation of T1 and T2 factors. The net effect of these events would be to retain isointensity within the area of the subacute infarct. Therefore, adding paramagnetic contrast to the region would be the only way of visualizing an abnormality on the basis of blood-brain barrier leakage of the agent.

References

1. McNamara NT, Brant-Zawadzki M, Berry I, et al. Acute experimental cerebral ischemia: MRI enhancement using Gd-DTPA. *Radiology* 1986;158:701–705.
2. Miyashita K, et al. Identification of recent lacunar lesions in cases of multiple small infarctions by magnetic resonance imaging. *Stroke* 1988;19:834–839.

Submitted by: Michael Brant-Zawadzki, M.D., Senior Editor.

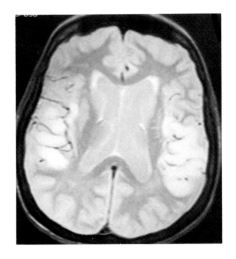

FIG. 83A. SE 2,800/35.

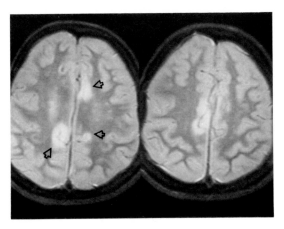

FIG. 83B. SE 2,800/35.

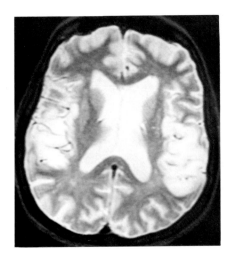

FIG. 83C. SE 2,800/70.

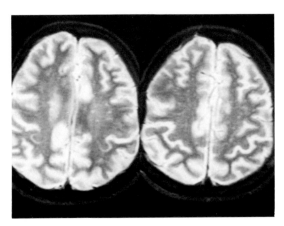

FIG. 83D. SE 2,800/70.

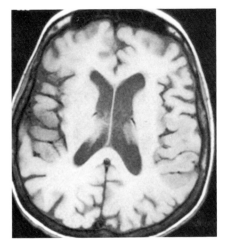

FIG. 83E. SE 700/20.

Clinical History

A 43-year-old woman with bilateral weakness and aphasia. The patient has a history of lupus.

Findings

Axial images at the level of the lateral ventricles and above using the T2-weighted technique (Figs. 83A–D) show homogeneous areas of high signal in the cortex of the middle cerebral artery distribution, as well as the anterior cerebral artery watersheds (Figs. 83B and D, *arrows*). Note the relative lack of mass effect of these lesions within the discrete vascular distributions mentioned. Also of interest is the fact that the lesions are more difficult to perceive on the second-echo images (Figs. 83C and D) given their isointensity with nearby cerebrospinal fluid. Note that the T1-weighted image (Fig. 83E) shows the area of abnormality as a subtle diminution of signal intensity.

Diagnosis

Systemic lupus erythematosus, multifocal arterial infarcts.

Discussion

A variety of clinical syndromes afflict the central nervous system in patients with systemic lupus erythematosus. The spectrum of changes includes sulcal enlargement, thought to be due to atrophy (or perhaps steroid use) through full-blown, territorial infarction. Vasculitis, in the strict sense of that term, is rarely, if ever, documented histologically in these patients. Marasmic endocarditis can produce embolic events as well. Patients with this disorder also harbor anticardiolipin antibodies in their serum, which predispose to recurrent arterial and venous thromboemboli.

The picture in this patient is that of classic arterial distribution infarction, with both middle cerebral artery territories affected. The anterior cerebral arteries show involvement in their watershed distribution.

References

1. Kaell AT, Shetty M, Lee BCP, et al. The diversity of neurologic events in systemic lupus erythematosus. *Arch Neurol* 1986;43:273–276.
2. Levine SR, Kim S, Deegan MJ. Ischemic stroke associated with anticardiolipin antibodies. *Stroke* 1987;18:1101–1106.
3. Levine SR, Welch K. Cerebrovascular ischemia associated with lupus anticoagulant. *Stroke* 1987;18:257–263.

Submitted by: Walter Kucharczyk, M.D., Toronto General Hospital, Toronto, Canada; Michael Brant-Zawadzki, M.D., Senior Editor.

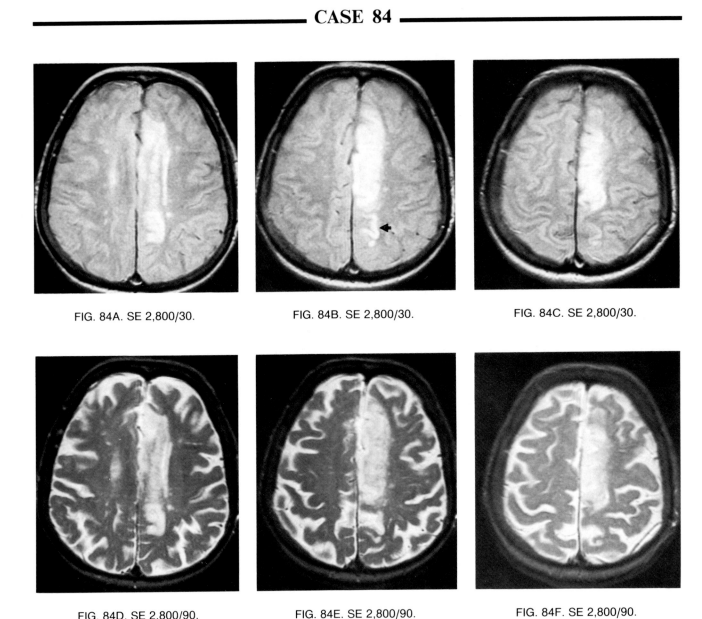

FIG. 84A. SE 2,800/30.

FIG. 84B. SE 2,800/30.

FIG. 84C. SE 2,800/30.

FIG. 84D. SE 2,800/90.

FIG. 84E. SE 2,800/90.

FIG. 84F. SE 2,800/90.

Clinical History

An 83-year-old woman with sudden onset of right leg weakness.

Findings

First echo (Figs. 84A–C) and second echo (Figs. 84D–F) images in the axial plane show a discrete area of increasing signal intensity in the paramedian frontal and parietal hemisphere immediately above the frontal roof. Note the predominant involvement of the gray matter, the relatively discrete margins of the lesion, and the gyriform distribution of the lesion in its posterior aspect (Fig. 84B, *arrow*).

Diagnosis

Anterior cerebral artery infarction.

Discussion

Isolated anterior cerebral artery infarction is rare, being seen in only 3% of all infarct cases. One of the reasons for this most likely relates to the relative pressure preferential flow into the cerebral artery in typical cases. Because embolic etiologies are responsible for most brain infarcts, the appearance of an anterior cerebral artery embolus should suggest the possibility of altered hemodynamics. For example, severe stenosis in a cervical carotid artery would prompt increasing flow into the anterior cerebral system from the contralateral carotid and a higher incidence of emboli into that system based on the higher flow volume. In addition, propagation of clot from an occluded internal carotid artery is a second mechanism whereby anterior cerebral artery infarction may occur. Finally, spasm, emboli, or propagating thrombosis associated with an anterior communicating artery aneurysm may predispose to these unusual types of infarcts.

Reference

1. Gacs G, Fox AJ, Barnett HJ, et al. Occurrence and mechanism of occlusion of the anterior cerebral artery. *Stroke* 1983;14:952–959.

Submitted by: Michael Brant-Zawadzki, M.D., Senior Editor.

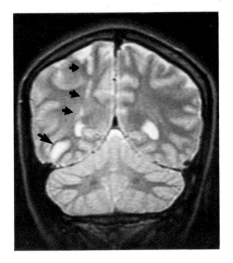

FIG. 85A. SE 3,000/70.

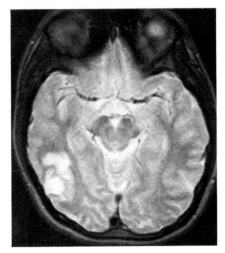

FIG. 85B. SE 2,800/70.

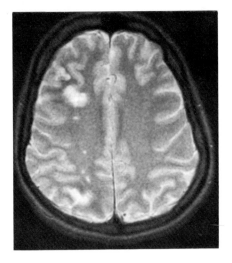

FIG. 85C. SE 2,800/70.

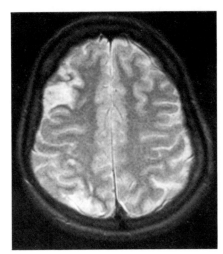

FIG. 85D. SE 2,800/70.

Clinical History

A 37-year-old woman with acute onset of headache, confusion, and nausea and vomiting.

Findings

The T2-weighted coronal (Fig. 85A) image documents high-signal foci throughout the deep right hemisphere (*arrows*) extending from the posterior temporal region up to the right parietal convexity. These foci are distributed in a curvilinear fashion. The axial views (Figs. 85B–D) demonstrate the lesions in a different plane. The larger foci of abnormality in the posterior right temporal, posterior right parietal, and midparietal region are accompanied by smaller foci (Fig. 85C) in the white matter.

Diagnosis

Watershed infarction, right middle cerebral artery.

Discussion

The distribution of lesions in this patient is quite typical for the "watershed" of the middle cerebral artery. This watershed region is the territory of the distal middle cerebral artery vessels where anastomosis with the anterior and posterior cerebral artery distribution occurs. In fact, this represents the farthest reaches of the middle cerebral artery system and includes the territories supplied by the deep perforating end vessels in the white matter and basal ganglia region.

In general, watershed infarction occurs due to hypoperfusion. As the hydrostatic force of flow recedes, the watershed regions are the first to be affected by the decrease in pressure. Obviously, emboli to the proximal trunks of the major vessels can produce watershed infarcts as well. Finally, microemboli can produce watershed infarction.

In summary, watershed infarcts are unique ischemic lesions that are situated along the border zones between the territories of the major cerebral arteries. Altogether, they constitute approximately 10% of all brain infarcts.

References

1. Torvik J, Ansgar A. The pathogenesis of watershed infarcts in the brain. *Stroke* 1984;15:221–223.
2. Wodarz R. Watershed infarctions and computed tomography. A topographic study in cases with stenosis or occlusion of the carotid artery. *Neuroradiology* 1980;19:245–248.
3. Sipponen JT. Visualization of brain infarction with nuclear magnetic resonance imaging. *Neuroradiology* 1984;26:387–391.

Submitted by: Michael Brant-Zawadzki, M.D., Senior Editor.

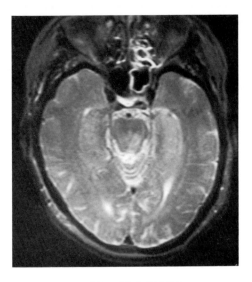 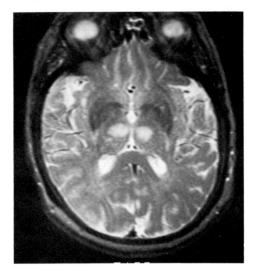

FIG. 86A. SE 2,800/90.   FIG. 86B. SE 2,800/90.

Clinical History

A 74-year-old woman with sudden onset of altered consciousness and leg weakness, and difficulty with eye movement, transient apnea, and amnesia noted on admission to the emergency room.

Findings

The two axial sections from the T2-weighted sequence demonstrate focal alteration of signal intensity within the thalamic nuclei bilaterally, as well as a subtle region of altered intensity in the left pontine tegmentum.

Diagnosis

Bithalamic infarction, embolic ischemic insult in the basilar artery distribution.

Discussion

Symmetric lesions within the thalamic nuclei, when associated with an acute syndrome such as the one described in the clinical history here, are somewhat typical for the "bithalamic syndrome" of amnesia, leg weakness, and altered state of consciousness. The typical inciting event is an embolic lesion. The arteriogram in this case demonstrated patency of the basilar artery (note the well-seen basilar artery in the lower section). However, the posterior cerebral arteries filled very slowly in their proximal segments, the distal distribution of the posterior cerebral arteries being slowly filled by collateral vessels from the middle cerebral arteries.

The relative lack of mass effect given to the lesions in an acutely ill patient and the localization of lesions to the basilar distribution (brainstem, thalami) are clues to the underlying etiology.

References

1. Bewerneyer H, Dreesbach HA, Rackl A, et al. Presentation of bilateral thalamic infarction on CT, MRI, and PET. *Neuroradiology* 1985;27:414–419.
2. Swanson RA, Schmidley JW. Amnestic syndrome and vertical gaze palsy: early detection of bilateral thalamic infarction by CT and MR. *Stroke* 1985;16:823–827.
3. Brant-Zawadzki M, Weinstein P, Bartokowski H. MR imaging and spectroscopy in clinical and experimental cerebral ischemia: a review. *AJNR* 1987;8:39–48.

Submitted by: Michael Brant-Zawadzki, M.D., Senior Editor.

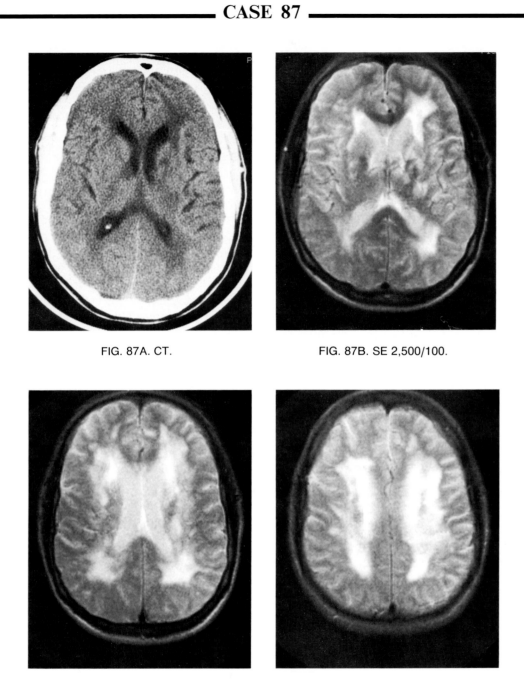

FIG. 87A. CT.

FIG. 87B. SE 2,500/100.

FIG. 87C. SE 2,500/100.

FIG. 87D. SE 2,500/100.

Clinical History

A 59-year-old man with altered mental status, nausea, vomiting, papilledema.

Findings

The CT scan (Fig. 87A) documents vague low-density regions within the periventricular area of the left frontal horn as well as in the caudate nucleus. T2-weighted axial images of the MRI study demonstrate diffuse high signal intensity in a patchy distribution throughout the deep hemispheric white matter, including the basal ganglia regions (left greater than right). Note the lack of mass effect as well as the ill-defined, spiculated borders of the patchy abnormalities and their nonspecific appearance.

Diagnosis

Hypertensive encephalopathy.

Discussion

The clinical presentation of hypertensive encephalopathy, related to sudden sharp increase in blood pressure, is that of severe headache, relentless nausea, vomiting, and confusion, possibly leading to stupor and coma. Papilledema and retinal hemorrhages are often found on eye examination.

Computed tomography studies in such patients have demonstrated low attenuation in cerebral white matter compatible with edema, progressing to compression of the ventricles, cisterns, and peripheral sulci in the more advanced cases. Typically, this is most evident in the supratentorial space. Reversal of such changes has been documented. Magnetic resonance imaging scanning, with its increased sensitivity to water in the brain, demonstrates to better advantage the altered signal intensity of the affected white matter resulting from the cerebral edema. Various etiologies have been suggested for the pathophysiologic changes occurring in hypertensive encephalopathy, including vascular spasm, breakdown of autoregulation of cerebral blood flow, and intravascular coagulation. Pathologic reports have documented fibrinoid necrosis of the small vessels and microinfarction with petechial hemorrhage. Therefore, a spectrum of mechanisms seemingly can produce the imaged abnormality.

The autoregulatory theory suggests that prolonged autoregulatory vasoconstriction in the face of high blood pressure causes spasm of these vessels, resulting in eventual arteriolar necrosis and abnormal permeability, which leads to full-blown edema and infarction. Reversibility in such cases would not be expected. This may be a partial mechanism for the chronic microangiopathic white matter changes seen in patients with long-standing hypertensive disease.

Another facet of this theory holds that with the autoregulatory vasoconstriction in the face of prolonged elevation of blood pressure, autoregulatory failure eventually occurs, producing total vasodilatation of the arterioles, with resulting hyperperfusion and hydrostatic "breakthrough" edema.

In any case, the typical changes are those shown here; namely, diffuse, relatively symmetric, white matter change that may resolve if it represents vasogenic edema and the hypertensive is treated aggressively. Obviously, if microinfarcts and even microhemorrhages occur in the course of this syndrome, reversibility would not occur, and MRI may show signs of blood by-products.

References

1. Rail DL, Perkin GD. Computerized tomographic appearance of hypertensive encephalopathy. *Arch Neurol* 1980;37:310–311.
2. Gibby WA, Stecker MM, Goldberg HI, et al. Reversal of white matter edema in hypertensive encephalopathy. *AJNR* 1989;10:S78.
3. Chester EM, Ajmanolis DP, Banker BQ, et al. Hypertensive encephalopathy: a clinical pathologic study of twenty cases. *Neurology* 1978;28:928–939.
4. Hauser RA, Lacey DM, Knight MR. Hypertensive encephalopathy: magnetic resonance imaging demonstration of reversible cortical and white matter lesions. *Arch Neurol* 1988;45:1078–1083.

Submitted by: Michael Brant-Zawadzki, M.D., Senior Editor.

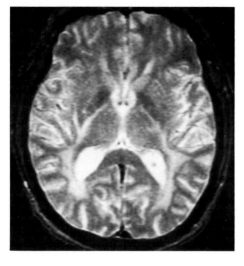

FIG. 88A. SE 2,800/70.

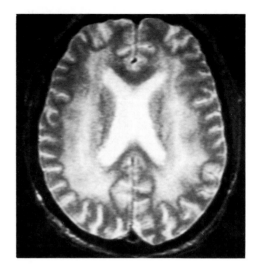

FIG. 88B. SE 2,800/70.

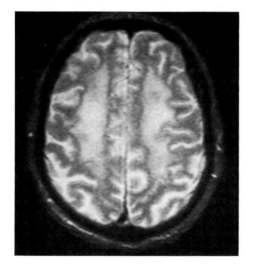

FIG. 88C. SE 2,800/70.

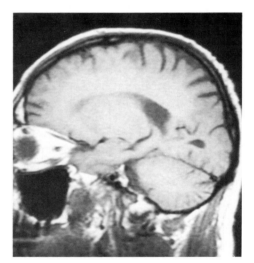

FIG. 88D. SE 600/20.

Clinical History

A 66-year-old patient with progressive dementia and a history of lymphoma and brain radiation.

Findings

The T2-weighted axial sequences (Figs. 88A and C) demonstrate diffuse alteration of the white matter with symmetric distribution throughout the centrum semiovale as well as the optic radiations (Fig. 88A), with involvement of the posterior external and internal capsules also noted. Of interest, the T1-weighted image (Fig. 88D) through the right hemispheric white matter is relatively unremarkable. Note the lack of either mass effect or atrophy.

Diagnosis

Radiation effect in cerebral white matter.

Discussion

A spectrum of central nervous system changes has been noted in the past on CT scans in patients due to whole-brain radiation, including atrophy, decreased attenuation of deep cerebral white matter, and focal, enhancing mass lesions due to radionecrosis. More recently, similar findings of radiation therapy-related lesions of the brain have been described with MR. Perhaps the most common is the diffuse elevation of signal throughout the hemispheric white matter, as shown in this particular case. The incidence of such changes appears to increase with advancing age, with only 20% of patients in the third decade of life showing them, compared with 82% in patients over the age of 60 years (1). In general, relative sparing of the brainstem, cerebellum, and internal capsules has been noted in this group of patients with diffuse white matter "pallor." The typical radiation dose ranged from 4,000–5,000 cGY. Chemotherapy may play a sensitizing role in these cases.

Magnetic resonance can also show focal radiation change much like the radionecrosis variant seen on CT. With breakdown of the blood-brain barrier due to small vessel disease produced by the radiation, contrast enhancement may occur in such cases.

References

1. Tsuruda J, et al. Radiation effects on cerebral white matter: MR evaluation. *AJNR* 1987;8:431–437.
2. Dooms G, et al. Brain radiation lesions: MR imaging. *Radiology* 1986;158:149–155.
3. Cavenes W. Experimental observations: delayed necrosis in normal monkey brain. In: Gilbert H, et al, eds. *Radiation damage to the nervous system.* New York: Raven Press, 1980;1–38.
4. Hecht-Leavitt C, et al. MR of brain radiation injury: experimental studies in cats. *AJNR* 1987;8:427–430.

Submitted by: Michael Brant-Zawadzki, M.D., Senior Editor.

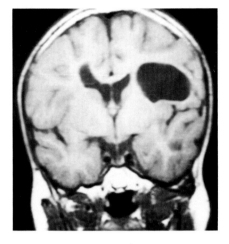

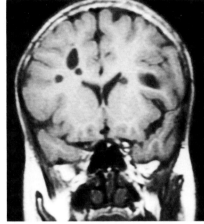

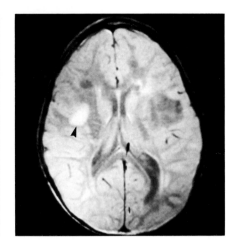

FIG. 89A. SE 600/20.

FIG. 89B. SE 600/20.

FIG. 89C. SE 2,500/35.

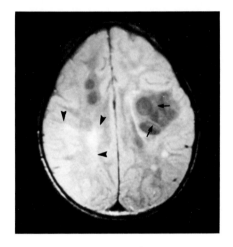

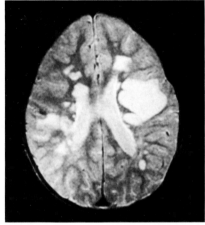

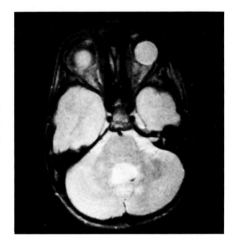

FIG. 89D. SE 2,500/35.

FIG. 89E. SE 2,500/70.

FIG. 89F. SE 2,500/70.

Clinical History

A 13-year-old boy with resection of cerebellar medulloblastoma 10 years previously and follow-up whole-brain and spine radiation therapy and chemotherapy.

Findings

Axial 5 mm T2-W (SE 2,500/35 and 70) and coronal 5 mm T1-W (SE 600/20) images are presented. There are multiple cystic lesions (Figs. 89A–E) scattered throughout both cerebral hemispheres, these changes being more prominent in the frontal regions and on the left side. Despite their size, none of these lesions appears to cause any significant mass effect. The largest lesion, in the left posterior frontal region, measures 4.5 cm in diameter, while the smallest lesions measure only 3–4 mm in diameter. The internal signal characteristics of these lesions parallels that of cerebrospinal fluid (CSF), although there are internal inhomogeneities and strands, best shown on the first echo of the T2-weighted sequence (Fig. 89D, *black arrows*).

There are upper lesions that do not parallel the signal intensity of CSF. These are of increased signal intensity on the first echo of the T2-weighted sequence and are both rounded (Fig. 89C, *arrowheads*) or more diffuse (Fig. 89D, *arrowheads*), the more diffuse component being predominantly in the white matter of the periventricular region and centrum semiovale. These lesions are not visible on the T1-weighted sequence. All of the abnormalities are centered in the white matter.

The 4th ventricle is enlarged, and there are mild patchy increases in signal intensity in the middle cerebellar peduncles and in the midline of the cortex of the left cerebellar hemisphere at the site of the previous resection (Fig. 89F).

Diagnosis

Radiation necrosis and postirradiation white matter ischemic changes.

Discussion

The multiple large cavities are the end result of radiation necrosis. These lesions tend to be more peripherally distributed in the white matter, as shown in this case, and initially are difficult to differentiate from tumor recurrence or other lesions, as acutely they have mass effect. However, as shown in this case, this mass effect resolves in time. The white matter ischemic disease is typically distributed more in the periventricular regions in the distribution of the long penetrating arteries. Radiation injury produces thickening and hyalinization in the walls of these vessels, resulting in a secondary ischemic injury, and accelerated deep white matter infarction is characteristic of patients who have undergone previous cranial irradiation.

The strands shown traversing the large cavity represent gliovascular bundles and may be seen pathologically in any brain cavity that results from brain necrosis (Fig. 89D, *arrows*).

Reference

1. Tsuruda JS, Kortman KE, Bradley WG, Wheeler D, VanDalsem W, Bradley TP. Radiation effects on cerebral white matter: MR evaluation. *AJNR* 1987;8:431–437.

Submitted by: Stephen J. Davis, M.D. and Louis M. Teresi, M.D., Huntington Medical Research Institutes, Pasadena, California; William G. Bradley, Jr., M.D., Ph.D., Senior Editor.

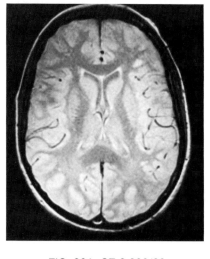

FIG. 90A. SE 2,800/30.

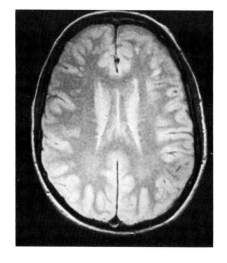

FIG. 90B. SE 2,800/30.

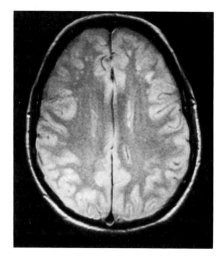

FIG. 90C. SE 2,800/30.

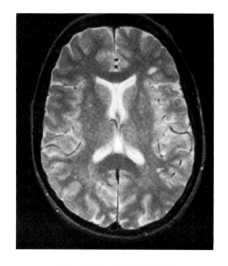

FIG. 90D. SE 2,800/70.

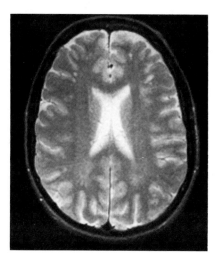

FIG. 90E. 2,800/70.

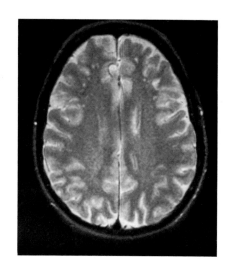

FIG. 90F. SE 2,800/70.

Clinical History

A 54-year-old woman with migraine headaches. Space-occupying lesion was suspected.

Findings

First echo (Figs. 90A–C) and second echo (Figs. D–F) consecutive axial sections through the brain reveal small foci of high signal intensity distributed in the subcortical white matter with no mass effect or surrounding edema. The higher cuts showed similar lesions distributed straight to the convexity.

Diagnosis

Presumed migraine-related ischemic changes in the brain.

Discussion

The lesions depicted here are a recently observed associated finding in patients with migraine syndrome. Forty-six percent of migraine sufferers demonstrated such lesions in a recent series. Any process that elevates the water content of the brain will prolong its T2 relaxation time and result in signal intensity elevation of the affected region. It is tempting to postulate that the lesions depicted here in association with migraine represent minute foci of ischemia due to spasm or possibly "breakthrough" edema from loss of autoregulation following a migraine attack. However, the real etiology for these lesions remains indeterminate. Frank infarction of large vessel branches has also been described with complex migraine attack.

Reference

1. Soges LJ, Cacayorin ED, Petro G, et al. Migraine evaluation by MR. *AJNR* 1988;9:452–459.

Submitted by: Michael Brant-Zawadzki, M.D., Senior Editor.

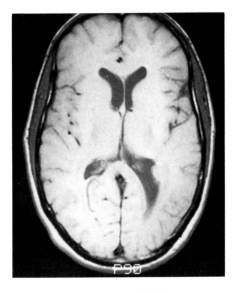

FIG. 91A. SE 800/20.

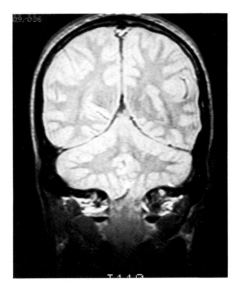

FIG. 91B. SE 2,800/30.

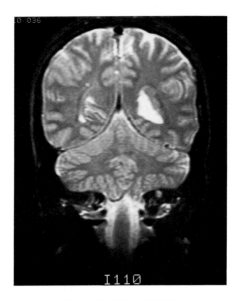

FIG. 91C. SE 2,800/80.

Clinical History

Seizures since childhood.

Findings

Lobulated mass is seen in the lateral aspect of the left ventricular trigone, both on the T1-weighted axial (Fig. 91A) and the dual-echo T2-weighted coronal (Figs. 91B and C) images. This mass shows signal intensity identical with that of normal gray matter, as shown on the T2-weighted coronal images. No surrounding edema is apparent, and the mass-like feature is evident only in relationship to the ventricular volume.

Diagnosis

Heterotopic gray matter.

Discussion

Periventricular masses can be due to a variety of causes. However, the most pathologic lesions will show signal intensity different from that of normal brain. When a lesion exhibits a signal intensity identical to that of gray matter, the entity of heterotopic gray matter is most likely.

The gray matter cortical mantle begins deep in the ventricular system and progressively migrates peripherally through uterine development. Occasionally, an arrest in this migration can occur, leading to the remnant foci of gray matter in the subependymal germinal matrix region. Small foci and, occasionally, large islands of gray matter may be seen. The clinical presentation is generally that of seizures, as in this case. Occasionally, overlying cortical mantle abnormalities may coexist, such as pachygyria.

References

1. Smith A, et al. Magnetic resonance imaging of disturbances in neuronal migration: illustration of an embryologic process. *Radiographics* 1989;9:509–522.
2. Barkovich A, et al. MR of neuronal migration anomalies. *AJNR* 1987;8:1009–1017.
3. Barkovich A, et al. Band heterotopias: a newly recognized neuronal migration anomaly. *Radiology* 1989;171:455–458.

Submitted by: Michael Brant-Zawadzki, M.D., Senior Editor.

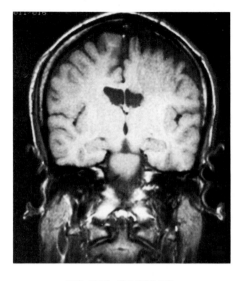

FIG. 92A. SE 600/20.

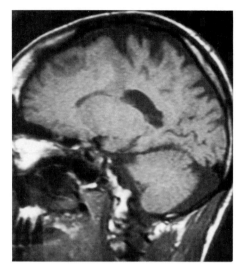

FIG. 92B. SE 600/20.

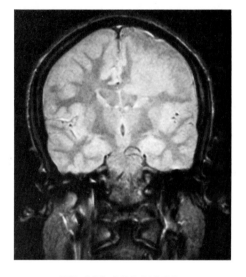

FIG. 92C. SE 2,800/30.

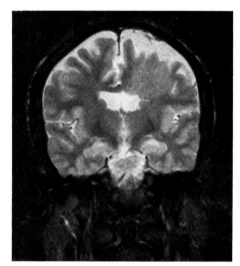

FIG. 92D. SE 2,800/70.

Clinical History

A 29-year-old man with long-standing seizure history and recent difficulty in control of seizures.

Findings

The T1-weighted coronal sequence (Fig. 92A) shows an asymmetry of the cerebral convexities, with the left parietal convexity showing an unusual gyral pattern typical of pachygyria: a relatively smooth-appearing cortical mantle with deformity of the gray-white interdigitation. Underlying this abnormality is a larger area of low signal intensity within the white matter (signal intensity matching that of gray matter) that extends all the way to the ventricular roof and indents it. This is shown to even better advantage on the sagittal T1-weighted image (Fig. 92B). The dual-echo coronal sequences again show this mass of tissue, which is isointense, with normal gray matter extending from the rather featureless cortical mantle through the white matter to the ventricular surface. Note that the intensity of this mass of tissue matches that of gray matter on both echos (Figs. 92C and D) of the T2-weighted sequence. Therefore, all three samplings of signal show the tissue to have the same signal intensity as gray matter.

Diagnosis

Gray matter band heterotopia with pachygyria.

Discussion

Incomplete neuronal migration from the subependymal germinal matrix to the cortical mantle results in various forms of gray matter heterotopia. Normally, during the 8th week of gestation, the neurons begin to migrate along radially oriented glial cells to predetermined, relatively distant final positions, where the cortical mantle forms. This process lasts two months, ending at approximately week 16. The cause of incomplete neuronal migration is unknown. Heterotopias have classically been separated into two forms. The nodular form consists of subependymal nodules of gray matter that are usually bilateral, although unilateral forms occasionally exist. The laminar form is seen as islands of gray matter that are usually isolated in the hemispheric white matter but may span the entire hemisphere between the ventricular surface and the cortex.

The 3rd form, band heterotopia, may constitute a form that is more difficult to identify because of the symmetric and diffuse nature of the anomaly. It is important to recognize that the thick band is isointense with gray matter and therefore does not represent abnormal white matter or a tumor mass. The relatively mild degree of pachygyria, which is unusual for such a severe migration anomaly, seems to coexist with the band type of heterotopia recently described.

Most patients with this disorder present with intractable seizures and developmental delay, although the development curve occasionally may be close to normal. However, the seizure problem is particularly difficult to control in such patients.

References

1. Barkovich A, et al. Band heterotopia of the gray matter. *Radiology* 1989;171:455–458.
2. Pinto-Lord M, et al. Obstructed neuronal migration along radio-glial fibers in the neo-cortex of the reeler mouse. *Dev Brain Res* 1982;4:379–393.
3. Taylor D, et al. Focal dysplasia of the cerebral cortex in epilepsy. *J Neurol Neurosurg Psychiatry* 1971;34:369–387.

Submitted by: Michael Brant-Zawadzki, M.D., Senior Editor.

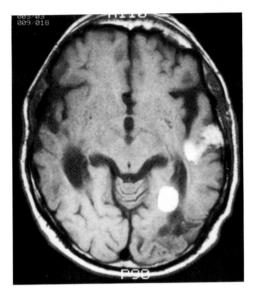

FIG. 93A. SE 700/20.

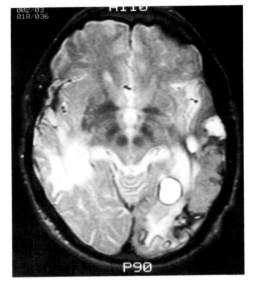

FIG. 93B. SE 2,800/70.

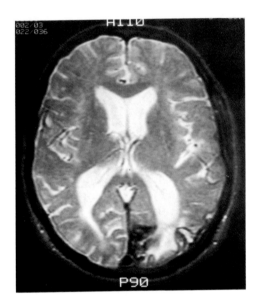

FIG. 93C. SE 2,800/70.

Clinical History

A 67-year-old man with a history of multiple cerebrovascular accidents.

Findings

T1-weighted axial study demonstrates two high-intensity lesions, one in the peripheral left temporal lobe and the second just underneath the left ventricular atrium (Fig. 93A). The T2-weighted sequences demonstrate both abnormalities as well as show serpentine areas of low signal in the posterior left temporal region and the right temporal periphery. The higher cut (Fig. 93C) demonstrates similar low signal intensity alteration of the calcarine region of the left occipital lobe.

Diagnosis

Multiple hemorrhages, underlying amyloid angiopathy.

Discussion

Cerebral amyloid angiopathy is caused by deposits of amyloid in the media and adventitia of small and medium-size arteries of the cerebral hemispheres, which are preferentially located in the superficial layers of the cerebral cortex and leptomeninges. It is virtually absent in the deep gray nuclei. This condition is restricted to the cerebrovasculature, as it is not associated with systemic vascular amyloidosis. This disease typically affects elderly individuals, its incidence in autopsy series increasing with age from a mere 8% in the 7th decade to close to 60% in individuals older than 90. The clinical result is intracerebral hematoma following rupture of an affected artery that is weakened due to the amyloid deposits. In short, microaneurysms can also result from such vessel wall weakening. Amyloid angiopathy is an important etiologic factor for spontaneous intracerebral hemorrhage in nonhypertensive elderly individuals, particularly those who present with recurrent hemorrhages of subcortical "lobar" location.

Magnetic resonance imaging quite nicely shows the residua of the older hemorrhages as preferential low signal intensity due to the hemosiderin staining of the previously damaged brain. The more recent hemorrhages show as either areas of methemoglobin-containing clot, seen as high signal intensity collection surrounded by edema (if fresh enough), or dioxyhemoglobin fresh bleeds.

Other possible causes of multifocal hemorrhages in various stages of evolution include familial occult arteriovenous malformations as well as metastatic foci (particularly from very hemorrhagic neoplasms, such as melanoma, hypernephroma, etc.).

References

1. Patel DV, Hier DB, Thomas CM, et al. Intracerebral hemorrhage secondary to cerebral amyloid angiopathy. *Radiology* 1984;151:397–400.
2. Tyler KL, Poletti CE, Heros RC. Cerebral amyloid angiopathy with multiple intracerebral hemorrhages. *J Neurosurg* 1982;57:286–289.
3. Kase CS. Intracerebral hemorrhage: non-hypertensive causes. *Stroke* 1986;17:590–595.

Submitted by: Michael Brant-Zawadzki, M.D., Senior Editor.

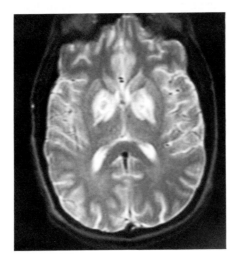 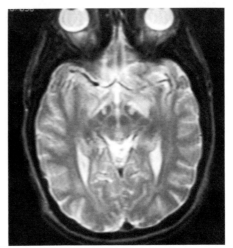

FIG. 94A. SE 2,800/80.   FIG. 94B. SE 2,800/80.

Clinical History

A 37-year-old white man who collapsed in his hotel room after snorting an unknown substance and who was unconscious for 30 hours. An MR scan was obtained nine days later.

Findings

Bilateral, symmetric lesions are seen in the lenticular nuclei (Fig. 94A) on the T2-weighted axial images shown. In addition, punctate focal lesions are present within the substantia nigra (Fig. 94B).

Diagnosis

Anoxic basal ganglia insults.

Discussion

Generalized anoxia can produce ischemic insult in the deep gray matter of the brain due to the selective vulnerability of these regions to any insult that deprives these highly metabolic foci of normal nutrients. Most commonly, insults of this nature are seen in diffuse hypoxia, carbon monoxide poisoning, or hypotensive ischemia. Given the history in this patient, that of drug abuse and subsequent coma (for 30 hours), the likeliest etiology is that associated with a global hypotensive episode, possibly drug induced. Surprisingly, this patient's mental status and neurologic function were essentially normal by the time this MR scan was obtained. More typically, global insults of this nature produce relatively profound neurologic deficits. For some poorly understood reason, this presentation of global anoxia/ischemia with preference for the basal ganglia tends to be seen more often in children and young adults than in older patients.

References

1. Takahashi S, Goto K, Fukasawa H, et al. Computed tomography of cerebral infarction along the distribution of the basal perforating arteries. *Radiology* 1985;155:107–118.
2. Brant-Zawadzki M, Weinstein P, Bartkowski H, et al. MRI imaging and spectroscopy in clinical and experimental cerebral ischemia: a review. *Am J Radiol* 1987;148:579–588.
3. Kjos BO, Brant-Zawadzki M, Young RG. Early CT findings of global central nervous system hypoperfusion. *AJNR* 1983;4:1043–1048.

Submitted by: Michael Brant-Zawadzki, M.D., Senior Editor.

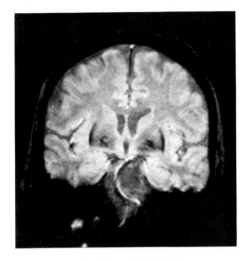

FIG. 95A. SE 800/15.

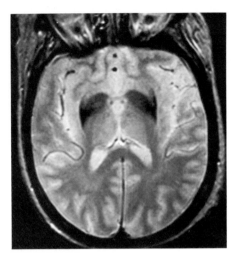

FIG. 95B. SE 2,800/45.

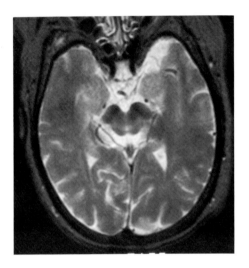

FIG. 95C. SE 2,800/90.

Clinical History

A 68-year-old man with shuffling gait and tremor.

Findings

The gradient-echo coronal (Fig. 95A) and dual-echo T2-weighted axial (Figs. 95B and C) images demonstrate lowered signal intensity within the putamen and substantia nigra. These are quite discrete abnormalities and conform to the structure involved rather than displacing or replacing it. No other definite abnormalities are shown.

Diagnosis

Parkinson's disease.

Discussion

Magnetic resonance studies of patients with Parkinson's disease have demonstrated a higher frequency of magnetic susceptibility effect within the globus pallidus, red nucleus, and substantia nigra, as well as the dentate nucleus. Iron may play an important role in neurotransmitter metabolism. It is postulated that in these regions, specific preferential T2 shortening results from local magnetic field heterogeneity produced by large molecules containing iron, such as ferritin and hemosiderin. Iron seems to be transported from other regions of the brain to regions of high iron content. When normal pathways are interrupted, increased iron accumulation may result.

There is a temporal sequence for normal increasing iron accumulation in these areas of the brain with advancing age. In general, decreased signal intensity in the basal ganglia and substantia nigra is not seen prior to the age of 25 years. However, severe ischemic/anoxic insults may produce changes similar to those produced by other forms of degenerative basal ganglial disease.

With advancing age, increasing iron accumulation may occur. Therefore, the diagnosis of Parkinson's disease based purely on the MR image of an elderly patient's brain is fraught with difficulty. Nevertheless, in a middle or early aged senior citizen, the finding of accentuated signal loss within the typical structure as described should raise the suspicion for the diagnosis of Parkinson's disease, particularly in the appropriate clinical setting.

References

1. Drayer B, et al. Magnetic resonance imaging of brain iron. *AJNR* 1986;7:373–380.
2. Drayer B, et al. Parkinson plus syndrome: diagnoses using high field MR imaging of brain iron. *Radiology* 1987;159:493–498.
3. Oaki S, et al. Normal deposition of brain iron in childhood and adolescence: MR imaging at 1.5T. *Radiology* 1989;172:381–385.
4. Dietrich R, et al. Iron accumulation in the basal ganglia following severe ischemic-noxic insults in children. *Radiology* 1988;168:203–206.

Submitted by: Roger Bird, M.D., Barrow's Institute, Phoenix, Arizona; Michael Brant-Zawadzki, M.D., Senior Editor.

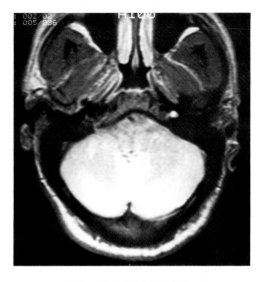

FIG. 96A. SE 2,800/30.

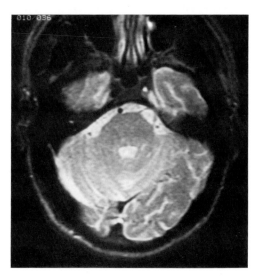

FIG. 96B. SE 2,800/70.

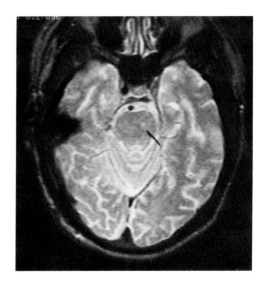

FIG. 96C. SE 2,800/70.

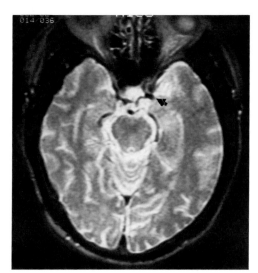

FIG. 96D. SE 2,800/70.

Clinical History

A 75-year-old man with left hemispheric transient ischemic attack.

Findings

The series of T2-weighted axial images from the base of the brain through the sella show an asymmetry in the course of the internal carotid arteries; specifically, the left internal carotid artery shows high signal seen in its petrous portion (Fig. 96A) that continues through to the cavernous portion (Fig. 96B), with the higher levels (Figs. 96C and D) not showing the large signal void present in the right internal carotid artery. Note the relatively normal appearance of the basilar artery, and the reasonably normal appearance of the supraclinoid tip of the left internal carotid artery (Fig. 96D, *arrow*). The angiogram (Fig. 96E) showed a highly stenotic precavernous segment of the left internal carotid artery, with marked cross-flow from the right, accounting for the washout of contrast from the intracranial left internal carotid artery circulation.

Diagnosis

Carotid occlusive disease.

Discussion

This case points out the sensitivity of MRI for the detection of highly stenotic or complete occlusive disease of the internal carotid artery system. Signal intensity within the high-flow carotid should be low on routine MRI sequences. When focal signal appears within this vessel, a high degree of stenosis or complete occlusion should be suspected. Nevertheless, it is difficult to distinguish between these two events, a critical point for patient management planning in the face of symptomatology. It remains to be seen whether the differentiation of a high degree of stenosis with slow flow, from complete occlusion, can be made with specific flow sensitive sequences being developed for MRI. It is likely that conventional arteriographic study will be necessary to differentiate these two entities.

Reference

1. Brant-Zawadzki M. Routine MR imaging of the internal carotid artery siphon: angiographic correlation with cervical carotid lesions. *AJNR* 1990. (In press.)

Submitted by: Michael Brant-Zawadzki, M.D., Senior Editor.

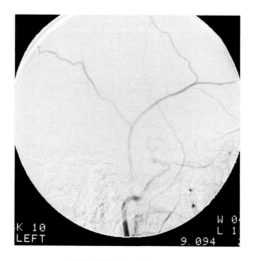

FIG. 96E. Angiogram.

221

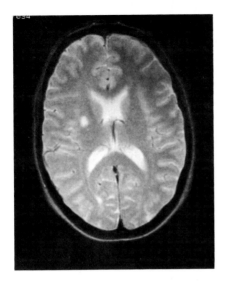

FIG. 97A. SE 2,500/70.

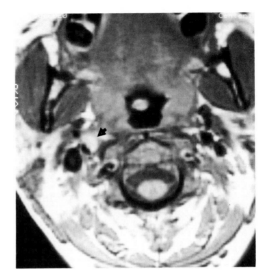

FIG. 97B. SE 1,400/20.

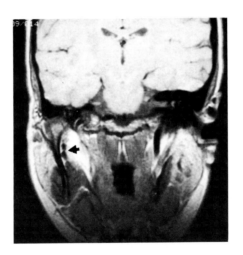

FIG. 97C. SE 1,000/20.

Clinical History

A 33-year-old aerobics instructor with sudden onset of left leg weakness following class, which resolved over six hours.

Findings

A 7 mm focus of high signal intensity is seen in the white matter of the deep right hemisphere on the T2-weighted axial image (Fig. 97A). The T1-weighted axial (Fig. 97B) and coronal (Fig. 97C) images demonstrate an abnormality of the right internal carotid artery in the neck. The axial image shows a compromise of its lumen, with only a small segment of signal void seen, compressed by a semilunar high-signal structure (Fig. 97B, *arrow*). The coronal image demonstrates a beaded appearance of this vessel (Fig. 97C, *arrow*) when compared with its counterpart on the left. The angiogram (Fig. 97D) verifies the presence of internal carotid artery dissection.

Diagnosis

Transient ischemic attack due to right internal carotid artery dissection, small infarct.

Discussion

The clinical point made by this case is that the patient's symptom was transient, the leg weakness resolving over six hours. Nevertheless, a permanent pathologic event occurred, as evidenced by the MR finding of a small infarct in the deep right hemisphere. It should be remembered that the term "transient ischemic attack" is a clinical entity, whereas the term "infarction" is a pathologic event. In fact, true pathologic infarcts can be completely silent. Therefore, it is not surprising that they can occur with the clinical presentation of a transient ischemic event as well as a permanent one.

In this case, the cause of the ischemic event was a spontaneous dissection of the internal carotid artery. Cervicocephalic arterial dissections are becoming recognized with increased frequency, particularly since the advent of MRI, which can identify these lesions non-invasively. Prior to this modality, angiograms might not have been done in many cases of dissections. However, with the findings depicted on the MR in this case, where the cervical carotid artery shows a clot in its wall compromising its lumen, angiography becomes mandatory. Demonstration of the cervical carotid dissection is generally followed by management with anticoagulants. In this way, more dire consequences, such as thrombosis and/or embolization distally, can be avoided. It should be noted that spontaneous resolution of dissection will occur in a substantial number of cases.

References

1. Biller J, Hingtgen WL, Adams HP. Cervicocephalic arterial dissections—a ten year experience. *Arch Neurol* 1986;43:1234–1238.
2. Pozzati E, Giuliani G, Poppy M, et al. Blunt traumatic carotid dissection with delayed symptoms. *Stroke* 1989;20:412–416.
3. Araki G, Mihara H, Shizuka M, et al. CT and arteriographic comparison of patients with transient ischemic attacks—correlation with small infarction of basal ganglia. *Stroke* 1983;14:276–280.

Submitted by: Michael Brant-Zawadzki, M.D., Senior Editor.

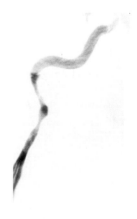

FIG. 97D. Angiogram.

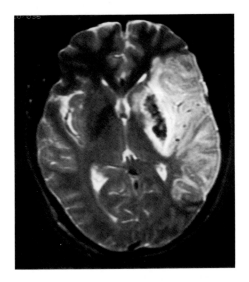

FIG. 98A. SE 2,800/90.

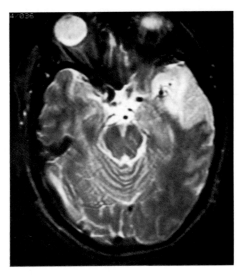

FIG. 98B. SE 2,800/90.

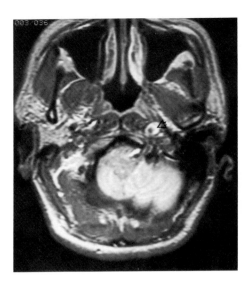

FIG. 98C. SE 2,800/30.

Clinical History

A 46-year-old businessman with sudden onset aphasia and right-sided hemiplegia. Onset came immediately after a throbbing headache. The patient has a history of hypertension.

Findings

T2-weighted axial images reveal a striking lesion in the distribution of the left middle cerebral artery, with high signal intensity in the cortex and subjacent white matter, but preferentially low signal intensity within the left basal ganglia (Figs. 98A and B). Note the asymmetry of the periclinoid carotid arteries with normal signal void within the right vessel but poor visualization of the left. The section obtained at the level of the foramen magnum reveals the left internal carotid artery with a collar of high signal intensity surrounding the low signal intensity center (Fig. 98C, *open arrow*). Selected views from the angiographic study document a dissection of the subcranial carotid artery with subsequent embolization into the internal carotid, anterior-middle cerebral artery system (Figs. 98D and E).

Diagnosis

Carotid artery dissection with subsequent left hemisphere infarction, complicated by secondary hemorrhage.

Discussion

Magnetic resonance imaging has greatly helped the early diagnosis of carotid vessel dissection by showing the hematoma within the vessel wall as high signal intensity constricting the low-signal lumen. In many cases in which the symptomatology is minor (acute headache, transient ischemic attack, etc.), the MRI can suggest the diagnosis and therefore prompt early angiography with subsequent anticoagulant treatment of the patient, which can prevent the dire consequences of this entity. With constriction of the lumen, thrombotic complications can occur with subsequent embolization and infarction into the brain, as had occurred in this case. Secondary hemorrhage into large middle cerebral artery infarction is well recognized in cases with major embolic events into the proximal and middle cerebral artery system; such hemorrhage is seen in up to 30% of cases. This occurs due to the fragmentation of the initial large embolus and subsequent reperfusion of the distally infarcted brain, with the force of systemic blood pressure applied to a disrupted autoregulatory mechanism within the distal vascular bed.

References

1. Goldberg HI, Grossman RI, Gomori J, et al. Cervical internal carotid artery dissecting hemorrhage: diagnosis using MR. *Radiology* 1986;158:157–161.
2. Pozzati E, Giuliani G, Poppy M, et al. Blunt traumatic carotid dissection with delayed symptoms. *Stroke* 1989;20:412–416.

Submitted by: Michael Brant-Zawadzki, M.D., Senior Editor.

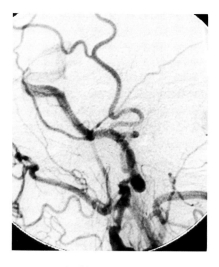

FIG. 98D. Angiogram.

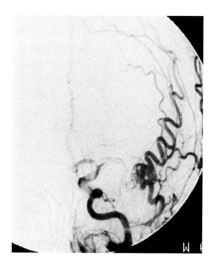

FIG. 98E. Angiogram.

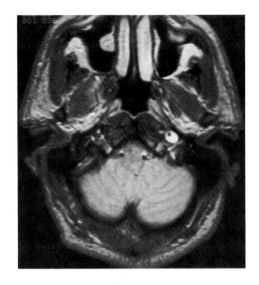

FIG. 99A. SE 2,800/30.

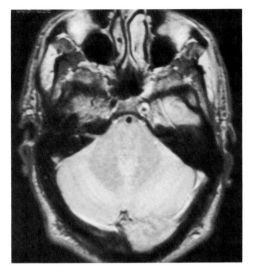

FIG. 99B. SE 2,800/30.

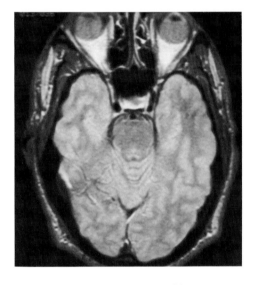

FIG. 99C. SE 2,800/30.

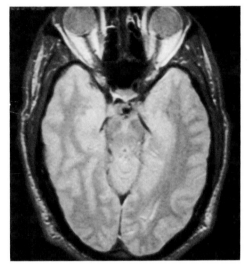

FIG. 99D. SE 2,800/30.

Clinical History

A 44-year-old man with sudden onset of left eye ptosis.

Findings

Axial sequences through the base of the skull and orbits (Figs. 99A–D) reveal no gross abnormality of the paracavernous region or the orbits. However, the lowest cut (Fig. 99A) shows a small signal void within the lumen of the internal carotid artery of the low petrous bone, with a high-signal collar surrounding it. This extends into the precavernous segment (Fig. 99B). Because of the combination of MR findings with the clinical syndrome, an angiogram was performed, verifying the suspicion of cervical carotid dissection (Fig. 99E).

Diagnosis

Carotid dissection.

Discussion

This is another example of carotid dissection, this time with the presentation of ptosis in the absence of any other symptomatology. The cause of ptosis in patients with carotid dissection relates to the disturbance of the occulosympathetic fibers to the sudomotor apparatus of the forehead, which travel along the internal carotid artery. Ptosis can be accompanied by the full-blown Horner's syndrome or the Raeder's variant.

Reference

1. Mokri B, Sundt TM, Houser OW. Spontaneous carotid artery dissection, hemicrania and Horner's syndrome. *Arch Neurol* 1979;36:677–680.

Submitted by: Michael Brant-Zawadzki, M.D., Senior Editor.

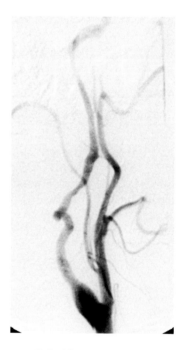

FIG. 99E. Angiogram.

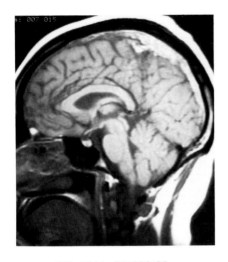

FIG. 100A. SE 800/20.

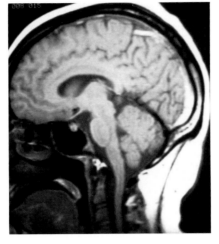

FIG. 100B. SE 800/20.

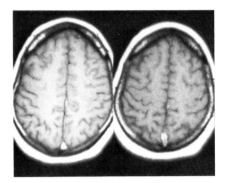

FIG. 100C. SE 600/20.

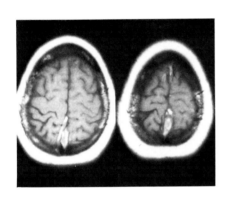

FIG. 100D. SE 600/20.

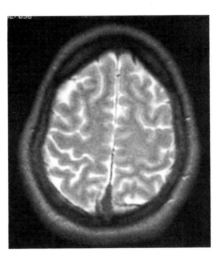

FIG. 100E. SE 2,800/90.

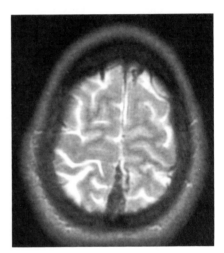

FIG. 100F. SE 2,800/90.

Clinical History

A 23-year-old woman with severe headaches for one week. Onset of dyplopia, nausea, and vomiting led to this MR scan one day later.

Findings

The T1-weighted sagittal sequences demonstrate high signal intensity within the general course of the sagittal sinus (Figs. 100A and B). The T1-weighted axial sequences verify this impression (Figs. 100C and D). The T2-weighted axial images (Figs. 100E and F) show the posterior sagittal sinus with preferentially lowered signal intensity within. No parenchymal abnormalities were noted.

Diagnosis

Sagittal sinus thrombosis.

Discussion

Thrombosis of the sagittal sinus (and other dural sinuses) can occur idiopathically or secondary to conditions such as pregnancy (in the puerperium), infection, trauma, malnutrition, dehydration, diabetes, a variety of hematologic disorders, including leukemia (particularly under treatment with L-aspariginase), and polycythemia vera. In general, the clinical symptomatology is that of elevated intracranial pressure, with papilledema and elevated pressure on lumbar puncture being the most common clinical signs. The prognosis is guarded with this condition; its recognition and institution of appropriate therapy (anticoagulation, either systemic or direct endovascular/transvenous) may ameliorate the condition. Consequences include hemorrhagic venous infarction due to extension of the occlusions to the cortical and transmedullary veins.

The MR appearance of the normal sagittal sinus is that of high-velocity signal loss on both T1- and T2-weighted sequences. Occasionally, flow phenomena, such as entry slice and second echo rephasing or pseudogating, can produce signal elevation within the dural sinuses on a fortuitously obtained image. Therefore, observation of the signal elevation on multiple images within a plane, as well as on acquisitions obtained in multiple planes, is important in excluding such phenomena as mimicking sinus thrombosis. It is important to note that clot with intracellular (red blood cell) deoxyhemoglobin or methemoglobin can show magnetic susceptibility effect-signal loss on T2-weighted sequences. This can simulate the normal signal void within a rapidly flowing sinus. However, the appearance of high-signal T1-weighted images of multiple sections, and the abnormal configuration of the sinus morphology in this case, clearly lead to the appropriate diagnosis.

Differential diagnosis includes midline lipoma of the intrahemispheric region. However, these lesions tend to be focal, round deposits rather than the curvilinear high signal intensity conforming to the sagittal sinus depicted here. Also, chemical shift phenomena can be helpful in identifying fat, as are fat suppression sequences.

References

1. Buonanno F. Computed cranial tomographic findings in cerebral sinovenous occlusion. *J Comput Assist Tomogr* 1978;2:281–290.
2. McMurdo S, et al. Dural sinus thrombosis: study using intermediate field strength MR imaging. *Radiology* 1986;161:83–86.
3. Nacchipj, et al. High field MR imaging of cerebrovenous thrombosis. *J Comput Assist Tomogr* 1986;10:10–15.
4. Bradley W, et al. Blood flow: magnetic resonance imaging. *Radiology* 1985;154:443–450.

Submitted by: Roger Bird, M.D., Barrow's Neurological Institute, Phoenix, Arizona; Michael Brant-Zawadzki, M.D., Senior Editor.

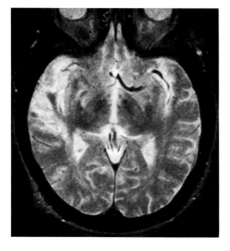

FIG. 101A. SE 2,800/70.

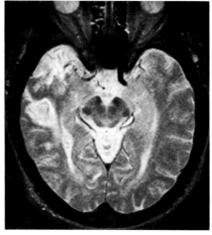

FIG. 101B. SE 2,800/70.

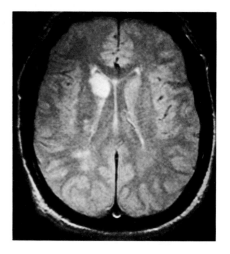

FIG. 101C. SE 2,800/30.

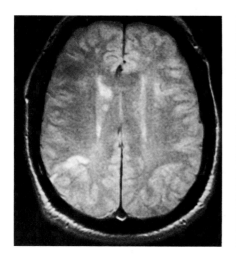

FIG. 101D. SE 2,800/30.

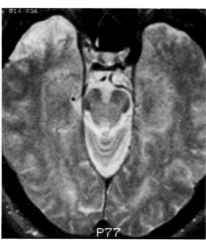

FIG. 101E. SE 2,800/70.

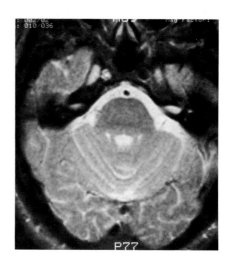

FIG. 101F. SE 2,800/70.

Clinical History

A 67-year-old man with fluctuating left leg paresis.

Findings

The T2-weighted, second echo images (Figs. 101A and B) show evidence of altered signal within the right temporal lobe and suggest narrowing in the right supraclinoid carotid artery (Fig. 101B). The first echo images from the same series demonstrate altered signal intensity in the caudate nucleus of the right hemisphere as well as the watershed region of the posterior right middle cerebral artery distribution (Figs. 101C and D). More precise evaluation of the cavernous right carotid artery on the second echo images (Figs. 101E and F) depict loss of the normal signal void when compared with the contralateral side. The subsequent angiogram (Figs. 101G and H) shows a "pseudo-occlusion" of the right internal carotid artery in the neck, with very slow antegrade flow of contrast depicted into the cavernous segment on the delayed (11 seconds) views.

Diagnosis

Right middle cerebral artery distribution infarction with "string sign" mistaken for complete right carotid artery occlusion on MR images.

Discussion

Routine MR images may strongly suggest high-grade occlusive disease or complete occlusion of a major intracranial vessel based on loss of the typical signal void seen within its lumen. However, without highly flow-sensitive techniques (and perhaps even despite their use), occasional instances of preocclusive disease, such as shown here, may be missed without conventional angiography being performed. This is an important management issue in that patients with this degree of occlusive disease may still be operable. In fact, surgery was performed in this case, with the very severely stenotic lesion responding to endarterectomy and reestablishment of flow in the internal carotid artery system on this side. Given the patient's mild symptoms and lack of global middle cerebral artery infarction, such an aggressive approach was chosen to avoid a further, larger infarct.

The parenchymal abnormalities shown here are quite typical for the appearance and distribution of middle cerebral artery branch infarction, including the perforator distribution to the basal ganglia.

Reference

1. Brant-Zawadzki M. Routine MR imaging of the internal carotid artery siphon: angiographic correlation with cervical carotid lesions. *AJNR,* August 1990.

Submitted by: Michael Brant-Zawadzki, M.D., Senior Editor.

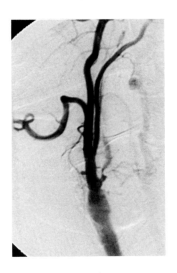

FIG. 101G. Angiogram.

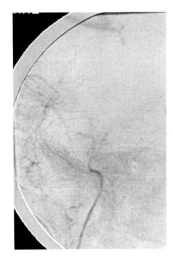

FIG. 101H. Angiogram.

NOTE: An *f* following a page number indicates an illustration.

236

239

Middle cerebral arteries
  aneurysm of, 152*f*, 153
  and infarction in systemic lupus erythematosus, 194*f*, 195
  left, aneurysm of, 154–155*f*, 155
  right
    aneurysm of, 156–157*f*, 157
    infarction in distribution of
    evolution of, 190*f*, 191
    "string sign" and, 230–231*f*, 231
    subarachnoid hemorrhage and, 180*f*, 181
    watershed, 198*f*, 199
Middle fossa, arachnoid cyst in, 122*f*, 123
Midline lesions, dysplastic, 164*f*, 165
Migraine headache, ischemic brain changes and, 208*f*, 209
Monro's foramen, ventricular reflux and, 159
Motion artifact, basilar artery pseudoaneurysm and, 170*f*, 171
Moyamoya, repeat intracerebral hemorrhage and, 29
Multiple telangiectasias, 52–54*f*, 55

N

Nausea
  in acute hematoma, 16, 17
  in hypertensive encephalopathy, 202, 203
  in lacunar infarcts, 18, 19
  in posterior inferior cerebellar infarcts, 8, 9
  in right middle cerebral watershed infarction, 198, 199
  in sagittal sinus thrombosis, 228, 229
Neonatal hemorrhages, in germinal matrix, 40*f*, 41
Neurinoma, resection of, dural thickening and, 166*f*, 167
Neurologic deficits, and arteriovenous malformations, with atrophy and hematomata, 86, 87
Newborn, subacute hematoma in germinal matrix in, 40*f*, 41
Numbness
  in cavernous angioma, 88, 89
  in hematoma and cortical siderosis, 44, 45
  in infarct and petechial hemorrhage, 190, 191
  in subarachnoid hemorrhage with infarction, 180, 181
Nystagmus, downbeat, and xanthogranulomata of choroid plexus and subfrontal meningioma, 96, 97

O

Obstructive hydrocephalus, 12
Occipital lobe, hemorrhagic infarction of, 34–35*f*, 36
Occulosympathetic fibers, carotid dissection affecting, 226–227*f*, 227
Occult arteriovenous malformations, 82*f*, 83
Osler-Weber-Rendu disease, 52–54*f*, 55
Oxyhemoglobin
  in acute subarachnoid hemorrhage, 160–161*f*, 161, 176–177*f*, 178–179
  in calcarine cortex hemorrhage, 34–35*f*, 36
  in hyperacute subdural hematoma, 130*f*, 131
  MR appearance of, 23
  persistent, within late subacute hematoma, 32*f*, 33

P-Q

Pachygyria, and heterotopic gray matter, 212*f*, 213
Papilledema, in hypertensive encephalopathy, 202, 203
Papilloma, of choroid plexus, 96*f*, 97
Paralysis. *See* Paresis
Paramagnetic contrast injection. *See also* Gadolinium contrast enhancement
  dural thickening illustrated with, 166*f*, 167
Parenchymal hemorrhage
  MR appearance of, 22–23
  repeat, 28*f*, 29
Paresis, and infarction in right cerebral artery distribution, 230, 231
Parietal arteriovenous malformation, and anterior communicating artery aneurysm, 64–66*f*, 67
Parietal lobes, atrophy of, 128*f*, 129
Parkinson's disease, 218*f*, 219
Pathologic hemorrhage, malignant glioma causing, 24*f*, 25
Periventricular region
  heterotopic gray matter in, 210*f*, 211
  shear injury affecting, 104*f*, 105
Petrous fracture, 106–107*f*, 108
Pial-dural arteriovenous malformations, 75
PICA. *See* Posterior inferior cerebellar artery
Polycythemia, sagittal sinus thrombosis in, 229
Pons
  hemorrhage in, 158–159*f*, 159
    acute to subacute, 162*f*, 163
    hypertensive, 51
  lacunar infarcts in, 18*f*, 19

Pontine syndromes, lateral inferior, and anterior inferior cerebellar territory infarct, 2*f*, 3
Porencephalic cyst, 128*f*, 129
Porencephaly, 127, 129
  posttraumatic, 128*f*, 129
Posterior cerebral arteries, adjacent interpeduncular branches of, infarct involving, 14*f*, 15
Posterior communicating artery, aneurysm of, 174*f*, 175
Posterior fossa
  hemorrhage originating in, ventricular reflux and, 159
  infarction in, mass effect and, 10–12*f*, 12
Posterior inferior cerebellar artery, infarction in distribution of
  acute, 8*f*, 9
  hemorrhagic, 4–6*f*, 7
Posterofrontal lobe, atrophy of, 128*f*, 129
Posttraumatic atrophy, 124*f*, 125
Posttraumatic edema, 110–111*f*, 112–113
  cortical, 146*f*, 147
Posttraumatic encephalomalacia, 124*f*, 125
  cystic, 132*f*, 133
  macrocystic, with calvarial defect, 126*f*, 127
Posttraumatic porencephaly, 128*f*, 129
Pregnancy
  and brain abnormalities in eclampsia, 188, 189
  sagittal sinus thrombosis in, 229
Pseudoaneurysm, basilar artery, motion artifact causing, 170*f*, 171
Pseudogating, diastolic, increased signal intensity and, 58
Ptosis, in carotid dissection, 226, 227
Pupillary sparing, in midbrain infarct, 14, 15
Putamen
  hypertensive hemorrhage in, 51
  infarct of, 16–17*f*, 17

R

Radiation necrosis, and postirradiation white matter ischemic changes, 206*f*, 207
Radiation therapy
  dural thickening and, 166*f*, 167
  white matter affected by, 204*f*, 205, 206*f*, 207
Raeder's variant, and disturbance of occulosympathetic fibers by carotid dissection, 227
Red nucleus, in Parkinson's disease, 218*f*, 219